Treating Individuals with Addictive Disorders

Integrating client stories, research and evidence-based strategies, this Workbook offers educational information, clinical tools and coping techniques to assist addiction patients on the journey toward recovery.

Chapters include psycho-educational information on the science behind addiction and examine how patients engaging in resilience behaviors can alter brain functions. A set of three appendices then evaluates what "works" for the treatment of individuals with addictive disorders including ways to engage patients in the treatment process and ways to assess residential treatment programs. Lastly, a glossary of the "language of recovery" terms provides patients and their family members with the guidelines to monitor treatment gains, support their journey of recovery and bolster their resilience.

Healthcare providers and those suffering from addictive disorders alike will benefit from the approachable discussion of the science and history behind addiction, the personal case-studies and the patient-friendly set of coping toolbox-activities designed to develop lasting behavioral changes.

Donald Meichenbaum, PhD, is one of the founders of cognitive behavioral therapy and he was voted "one of the ten most influential psychotherapists of the 20th century.' He has consulted at Addiction Treatment Centers for thirty years.

Treating Individuals with Addictive Disorders

A Strengths-Based Workbook for Patients and Clinicians

Donald Meichenbaum

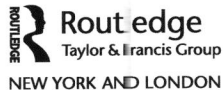
Routledge
Taylor & Francis Group

NEW YORK AND LONDON

First published 2020
by Routledge
52 Vanderbilt Avenue, New York, NY 10017

and by Routledge
2 Park Square, Milton Park, Abingdon, Oxon, OX14 4RN

Routledge is an imprint of the Taylor & Francis Group, an informa business

Library of Congress Cataloging-in-Publication Data
Names: Meichenbaum, Donald, author.
Title: Treating individuals with addictive disorders : a strengths-based
    workbook for patients and clinicians / Donald Meichenbaum.
Description: New York, NY : Routledge, 2020. | Includes bibliographical
    references and index.Identifiers: LCCN 2020002695 | ISBN 9780367440305
    (hardback) | ISBN 9780367440282 (paperback) | ISBN 9780367440282 (ebook)
Subjects: LCSH: Substance abuse—Treatment—Handbooks, manuals, etc. |
    Substance abuse—Psychological aspects—Handbooks, manuals, etc.
Classification: LCC RC564.15 .M45 2020 | DDC 616.86/06—dc23
LC record available at https://lccn.loc.gov/2020002695

ISBN: 978-0-367-44030-5 (hbk)
ISBN: 978-0-367-44028-2 (pbk)
ISBN: 978-1-003-00717-3 (ebk)

Typeset in Helvetica & Garamond Three
by Swales & Willis, Exeter, Devon, UK

This book is dedicated to the many clinical staff who have provided me with an opportunity to consult at their treatment facilities. It is also dedicated to their patients who have provided constructive feedback on the Coping Exercises included in this Patient Workbook. In particular, I wish to acknowledge the contributions of Lawna Anderson and Julie Myers for their collaborative work on relapse prevention triggers and SMART Recovery, respectively. In addition, a special thank you goes to Candace and Michael Lowry, Roy Cameron and Lise Perrin-Gleissle, who have supported my clinical consultations at their settings. Finally, this book is dedicated to the memory of Alan Marlatt, who was a pioneer in the treatment of individuals with Addictive Disorders.

Table of Contents

Prologue

If you, or a loved one, is addicted to alcohol, or drugs like opioids, or have a behavioral addiction like gambling, sex, eating or computer use, there is a way to achieve "lasting changes." There is hope!

This book provides accounts of individuals who have recovered from addictions and the specific steps they took to develop a Coping Tool Box and nurture their resilience. As a result of reading this book and doing the suggested Exercises you will be able to:

1. develop a better understanding of how addictive behaviors and mental health issues affect the brain and other bodily functions, and social relationships ("*How the body keeps score*");
2. how you can build upon your strengths and resilience and use your positive emotions and thinking processes to reshape your brain and behaviors and help you achieve your treatment goals ("*The brain is malleable and adaptable*");
3. learn ways to self-regulate cravings and urges, self-soothe and tolerate negative emotions, reduce both your stress level and cue sensitivity, improve your Coping Tool Box, and build and broaden positive emotions;

   "*Addiction is the experience of losing control over oneself*";

4. learn how to use relapse prevention skills that contribute to "lasting changes" ("*The question is not only why the addiction, but why the pain*");
5. learn how to develop and maintain a social network of people who support abstinence and your personal journey of recovery and well-being;
6. develop a *sobriety script* and specific doable plans in order to sustain a balanced life-style;
7. share what you have learned and deliberately practiced with significant others, making a "gift" of your experiences, using the language of recovery.

This Patient Workbook provides a *strengths-based* approach that focuses on how individuals can achieve and maintain treatment gains and develop rewarding drug-free activities and relationships that sustain recovery. The table of contents lists the personal Exercises you can do in order to use your recovery resources, foster hope by highlighting the benefits of behavior change and increase the likelihood of your reducing substance abuse and you becoming abstinent.

This book is written for both individuals who are currently receiving treatment for addictive disorders and co-occurring psychiatric disorders and for individuals who want to take actions to change. Family members of individuals who have addictive behaviors will also find this book of value.

The Stories We Tell Ourselves

We each are not only homo-sapiens, but we are also "homo-narrans", or story-tellers. We each tell ourselves, and others, stories designed to explain our behavior and accompanying feelings, as well as the choices and decisions we make. In short, we are lived by the stories we tell ourselves and the narratives we offer others.

This applies, especially to the addictive behaviors individuals choose to engage in. Whether it is the use of alcohol or drugs, pathological gambling, compulsive eating or sexual addictions, an individual's thinking processes in the form of the reasons, rationalizations and denials sustain such addictive behaviors.

This book traces the accounts and stories of how individuals with addictive behaviors develop "recovery" narratives and the accompanying coping behaviors to become abstinent. Consider the following accounts, as noted below, that illustrate this transition from addiction to recovery. This is followed by nine modules that provide practical user-friendly Exercises on ways to redirect your narrative and develop an accompanying Coping Tool Box in order to change your addictive behaviors.

We begin Module I with a consideration of illustrative thinking processes (story-telling) that sustains addictive behaviors. This negative mindset results in "Addiction Traps". Telling yourself and others the following increases the likelihood you will become or stay addicted.

"I am stuck in a negative mindset."

"My life is destroyed already. There is nothing worth saving."

"I feel – trapped, stuck, powerless, shattered, hollow, ashamed, guilty, angry, insecure."

"Alcohol/drugs has hijacked my brain."

"I am locked in a battle and cannot win."

"I feel paralyzed. I shut down and gave up. I feel doomed."

"I am detached from my inner life, a burden on others and a complete failure."

"The weight of my past made me make bad decisions."
"The drinking (drug use) became a way to shut down my feelings."
"I do not have a history of addiction in my family."
"I am addicted to the allure of the life-style."
"I just love the highs and the rush."
"I cannot face the withdrawal symptoms, so I have to continue using."

In addition to these examples of a negative mindset, addicted individuals also have the ability to play mind games and engage in "twisted thinking", as discussed in Module V. As the adage notes:

"Alcoholism is 10% drinking and 90% thinking."

This Patient Workbook highlights the 90% thinking processes and how to move from a Negative Addictive Mindset to a Positive Recovery Mindset. The good news is that Substance Abuse Disorders are highly treatable. A majority of affected individuals do recover.

In contrast, consider the voices and accounts of individuals who become abstinent and are in recovery. Their story-telling usually includes the following features:

1. Some reference to being on a personal journey, and is usually filled with change talk and the language of possibility, as discussed in Module V. For example:

    "I am in the midst of a transformation."
    "I now have hope. I can envisage who I might become. A new possible self."
    "I now have a guiding light. I can follow my faith."
    "I recognize that recovery is hard work and it requires effort and patience."
    "I learned to do things outside my comfort zone."
    "I learned to look beyond my negative emotions and cravings to positive outcomes that lie ahead."

2. Individuals in recovery also refer to a variety of coping skills that they use in response to various personal and interpersonal challenges such as triggers to use, cravings, negative emotions, interpersonal conflicts and social pressures and stressors. As to be discussed in the modules below, these coping skills cover behavioral, emotional, cognitive, interpersonal and spiritual domains.

"I can now surf my urges and become curious about them."
"I learned to dialogue with my urge. What did my urge want me to get away from?"
"I learned to quiet my inner critic."

Recovery is not something that is reached or achieved. Recovery is fluid, dynamic and diverse. Recovery is filled with new beginnings.

This book is a detailed description of how individuals move from a negative mindset to have a resilient coping repertoire that sustains their recovery. Each of the following Exercises provide guidelines on how to begin to redirect your narrative and develop and implement your Coping Tool Box.

You can visit the following Websites to hear the accounts ("stories") that individuals who are in recovery offer to others and to themselves. This book provides ways in which you can join this recovery group and improve your well-being and become abstinent.

Listen to Elizabeth Vargas, who was an ABC television anchor, tell her battle with alcohol and the road to recovery **abcnews.go.com/Health/ abc-news-anchor-Elizabeth-Vargas**

Here are several other Websites that you can call up in order to listen to their Recovery stories.

www.crisisnextdoor.org
www.storiesofrecovery.org.uk/index.php
www.recoverymonth.gov/personal-stories/read
www.ncadd.org/people-in-recovery/recovery-stories
www.heretohelp.bc.ca/personal-stories

In addition, see the recently published book "Never enough: The neuroscience and experience of addiction" by Dr. Judith Grisel, who is a neuroscientist and a professor at Bucknell University in Pennsylvania. She tells the poignant story of how she went from being a major drug addict to being sober for thirty years and what contributed to her productive life of abstinence. I will share her story and observations throughout this Patient Workbook. Also included are **discovery voices** of individuals who have used these Exercises in their Journey of Recovery.

At the end of each module are a series of quotations that summarize that module's main points. These quotes should be considered as a form of ***discussion starters*** that you can share with others, or that you can reflect upon by yourself. They are a kind of "*brain teasers*" that underscore the message of the Exercises that are included in that module. In addition, included at the end of this Patient Workbook (on pages 188 to 203) is a **glossary** of terms that will help you develop and use the "Language of Recovery".

DISCUSSION STARTERS FOR MODULE I

"We become the stories we tell about ourselves. Beware of the stories you tell yourself and that you tell others."

"Humans are natural story-tellers. The stories we tell ourselves and tell others influence the lives we live."

"We are what we pretend to be, so we must be careful about what we pretend," (Kurt Vonnegut, "Mother Night").

"It is not heroin, alcohol, nicotine or cocaine that makes an addict. It is the drive to escape from reality. Chemicals are not the only way to escape. Some become behavioral addicts of the internet, pornography, sex, food, shopping and work." Neuroscientist Judith Grisel

RECOVERY VOICE I: MY CHILDHOOD HERO

I am known as a polysubstance abuser. Name a drug, and I have used it. I have been in and out of several Treatment Centers. My current therapist gave me this Patient Workbook and encouraged me to look up the Websites listed of addicts who have recovered. I was reluctant to do so, since I have sat through numerous AA meetings and listened to multiple "drunk-a-logs". In order to please her, I clicked on the Website www.crisisnextdoor.org. Lo and behold, there was my childhood hero, the famous baseball player and his wife – Darryl Strawberry telling their story of woe and recovery from addiction.

Strawberry was a phenomenal ball player. (Google him and his Rehabilitation Institute.) I have carried his baseball card with me to this day. Whenever I have the urge to use drugs again, I take out his baseball card, and it helps me maintain my sobriety.

In fact, I have now listened to other Recovery Stories on the Websites and those listed in this Patient Workbook. I have become an "exquisite listener" to how these recovered addicts have incorporated **Change Talk** into their journey stories of recovery.

My childhood hero is still influencing my behavior. Another RBI (Run Batted In) for Strawberry.

These patient accounts are very moving. As a collection, they are inspiring, reflecting a complex portrait of resilience. The result is not just a fascinating read, but an important testimonial. I encourage you to read each of the many Recovery Stories. There is hope!

Psycho-Education

What You Need To Know

Exercise 1: Some Basic Information About Addiction: Vulnerability Factors

Exercise 2: How the Brain Gets Addicted: Implications for Recovery

Exercise 3: The "Body Keeps Score" of Both Negative and Positive Effects: Ways to Reshape Your Brain

Exercise 4: Understanding the Connection Between Feelings, Thoughts and Behaviors: Use of a "Clock" Metaphor

Please see the YouTube video by Dr. Judith Grisel: "Never enough: The Neuroscience and Experience of Addiction" for a very informative presentation.

One of the main objectives of this Patient Workbook is to help patients make *informed decisions* and *healthy choices*. This module begins with a discussion of basic information about the nature and impact of addictive behaviors and *vulnerability* factors that predispose individuals to become addicted (Exercise 1).

This is followed by a discussion of "How the brain gets addicted", and the implications for recovery (Exercise 2).

The *good news* is that with your efforts, and the support of a Treatment Team, you can *reshape your brain* and begin to achieve your treatment goals. How you can build and broaden your *positive emotions* and engage in *resilience-engendering behaviors* to develop new neural pathways and adaptive-behaviors are the focus of Exercise 3.

Exercise 4 will highlight the ways that your feelings, thoughts, behaviors and the reactions of others, are all *interconnected*. A simple Clock metaphor will be presented so you can better analyze any situations you will encounter. In fact, you will be able to *teach* this Clock analytic tool to others in your life.

As a result of completing this module, you will be better prepared to benefit from the remaining modules in this Patient Workbook that focus on collaborative goal-setting (Module III), ways to improve your Coping Tool Box for handling your emotions (Module IV), your thinking processes (Module V) and your social relationship (Module VI).

You will be able to explain, to others in your life, how some people become addicted to substances and the impact it has had on their lives, and most importantly, what it takes to recover, become abstinent and improve one's quality of life. You will also be able to provide the *reasons* why doing so is important.

As you work through the remaining modules, you will be able to describe and use the specific Coping Tools you have developed that will help you in your personal journey toward abstinence and well-being. I suggest that you acquire a loose-leaf book of pages and label the book "My Recovery Voice". You can use this book to do the various Exercises in this Patient Workbook.

EXERCISE 1
SOME BASIC INFORMATION ABOUT ADDICTION: VULNERABILITY FACTORS

Substance abuse disorders affect some 14% of the U.S. population in any given year. We begin with a consideration of the vulnerability factors that contribute to developing such addictive behaviors. Research indicates that a variety of factors including one's inheritance, exposure to childhood adversities, early substance abuse, as well as one's current level of toxic stress and accessibility to substances, each combine to determine an individual's vulnerability to develop addictive behaviors. Let us briefly consider each source of factors.

In terms of inheritance, some children are dealt "a set of genetic cards, or a bad hand", when they are born that render them vulnerable to develop addictive behaviors. They are up against the odds. Addictions tend to run in families and a transmittable genetic loading may be passed from one generation to the next. For example, a family history of alcoholism increases the risk of offspring developing a similar proclivity by three to five times, as compared to those who do not have such a family addicted behavior. Children of addicted parents respond differently to the ingestion of alcohol with increased elation, pleasure and relaxation, and with decreased feelings of intoxication when they ingest alcohol and various other drugs later in life. An inheritable risk factor for alcohol dependence is tolerance and a relative insensitivity to alcohol, or the ability to "hold your liquor" without feeling or appearing to be affected by alcohol as others are.

Children of alcoholic parents have higher levels of serotonin in their bodies and when they ingest alcohol this predisposes them to develop an increased vulnerability to become addicted that contributes to a number of psychological and behavioral levels of anxiety, depression and aggression. In addition, they have the penchant to engage in the usage of other addictive substances (polysubstance use).

Further evidence of the role of heritability comes from studies of identical twins who have the exact same genetic makeup, as compared to fraternal twins who *do not* share the same genetic makeup. The identical twins have a higher concordance rate and incidence of substance abuse than do fraternal twins.

> It is estimated that up to 50% to 60% of risk for developing addiction is due to heritability.

The fact that substance abuse disorder is partly heritable only tells you about population-level transmission, but it does not tell whether a particular person will inherit the disorder. No psychological trait or behavioral disorder is 100% heritable. For instance, it is worth noting that even though identical twins share a 100% DNA genetic composition, only some 50% of the identical twins go on to develop addictive disorders. This means that other factors contribute to vulnerability to developing addiction, such as the exposure to recurrent Adverse Childhood Experiences (ACE).

Such vulnerability to developing addictions is exacerbated if the child also has been exposed to *recurrent early* ACE such as physical, sexual and emotional abuse, and various forms of neglect and/or exposure to school, family and community violence.

The *pile-up* of *four or more* such ACE have been found to increase the likelihood of becoming addicted to alcohol and other drugs by *500 times*, *versus* those individuals who did *not* experience such adverse childhood events. Exposure to multiple adverse childhood events can sabotage brain development, especially in the impulse control areas that do not fully develop. This can lead to a *hair-trigger* response to events and conversations that other people just shrug off. These ACE events are biologically embedded in your body and can "wear and tear" on the body.

Individuals who have six of more ACE scores have a fore-shortened life-span of up to twenty years. As we will consider, if you have a high ACE score, *you are not* doomed.

> "One's history is not one's destiny. The brain is very plastic and the body wants to heal."

Such developmental adverse influences can be further exacerbated if an individual *begins substance abuse during early adolescence*, as part of an association with a peer group who also uses substances (smoking, alcohol, marijuana and "hard" drugs), in part due to low parenting monitoring. The earlier the onset of substance use, the greater the vulnerability to develop adult addictive behaviors. Early use renders the brain to become dependent on substances. People who do not begin drinking, smoking or using illicit drugs before age 21 are much *less likely* to develop disabling addictive disorders in adulthood.

For each year before age 21 that individuals begin using substances, they increase the likelihood of developing an adult substance abuse disorder by 7%. Thus, if individuals begin using substances by ages 12 or 13, they increase their risk by some 70% to 80%. If individuals delay using substances like alcohol to their mid-twenties, when the brain has matured, they are likely to only become social drinkers, rather than develop some form of addictive disorder.

Early substance abuse, especially when the brain is developing and before it fully matures, causes neural changes that increase the likelihood of problematic, addictive behaviors in adulthood. Such early copious use of substances undermines the development of the prefrontal cortex resulting in impulsive behaviors, and deficits in both abstract thinking and the ability to delay gratification. Early use of substances results in individuals being four times more likely to eventually meet the criteria of substance abuse disorder.

Early usage of substances is associated with children and youth who evidence a disorder of hyperactivity. Attention Deficit Hyperactivity Disorder (ADHD) may co-occur with a variety of other disorders such as Oppositional Defiant Disorder (ODD) and Conduct Disorder (CO). These compounding behavioral changes contribute to deficits in emotional self-regulation and poor "top down" inhibition, a difficulty in exerting executive (frontal lobe) functioning resulting in impulsive rapid decision making with a preference for immediate gratification and a discounting of delayed negative consequences. They also evidence a diminished ability to self-monitor and less self-awareness. Individuals who are prone to be impulsive and engage in sensation-seeking activities, and seek novelty, who are not swayed by punishment or negative consequences, are more vulnerable to use various substances. In summary, a variety of developmental factors that reflect deficits in self-regulation in childhood and adolescence predict later onset of Substance Abuse Disorders. These include a difficult temperament, and conflicts with authorities and the law. This pattern of behavior predisposes them to develop substance abuse disorders as they enter early adulthood.

But it is *not* only early stress that can contribute to addictive behaviors, but also exposure to chronic toxic ongoing stress during adulthood. In fact, some addictive individuals, experience what is called a "double whammy". They not only have problems of struggling with their addiction, but this may be complicated by the occurrence of some form of mental disorders. Such mental disorders may precede, accompany or follow the onset of addictive disorders. Such co-occurring disorders require a comprehensive integrated treatment approach.

> "I learned how my trauma history and addictive behaviors are related."

The exposure to chronic toxic stress leads to the body's continuous response of adrenaline and cortisol secretion that increases blood pressure and can, in turn, impact the circulatory system. The use of addictive substances to cope with such stressors only makes things worse by stimulating the parasympathic nervous system that further contributes to the wear and tear of the body. Thus, a "vicious cycle" develops between vulnerability factors, exposure to a life-time of adverse

events and ongoing experience of stress. People may use substances to break this vicious cycle in a form of *self-medication*.

Some heavy drinkers, or individuals who use addictive drugs, can stop and change their behaviors on their own, but many need professional help, especially if they use several different drugs in addition to alcohol, and if they experience multiple psychiatric disorders. These factors are further exacerbated by high availability of drugs and alcohol. If the use of substances are part of a cultural norm and expectancy, then this too can contribute to addictive behaviors.

Take some time to discuss with your Treatment Team what factors may have contributed to your vulnerability to develop addictive disorders, and any co-occurring disorders you may experience. Did heritability, early childhood aversive experiences, early usage, ongoing exposure to chronic stress, social pressure and cultural expectations play a role in your present difficulties? What other factors may have contributed to your presenting problems?

> It is what happened to you, not what is wrong with you that is the critical question, and what can you do to change?

EXERCISE 2
HOW THE BRAIN GETS ADDICTED: IMPLICATIONS FOR RECOVERY

About three in ten adults drink at levels that elevate their risk of developing alcoholism, with accompanying liver disease and an array of other physical, mental and social problems. For adults who exceed the low risk level of four drinks on a given day, and seven drinks a week, one in four will become an alcoholic. The level of risk increases if the individual is a polysubstance user (combines alcohol with other substances such opioids, heroin, cocaine, marijuana, tobacco).

If individuals drink too quickly, or if they have certain medical problems, or are older, they are predisposed to become addicted.

Chronic alcohol and other substance abuse contribute to increased level of stress, anxiety, depression, and most importantly, interfere with sleep behavior, causing insomnia, loss of deep sleep and recuperative REM (rapid eye movement) sleep that are needed for a restful night's sleep.

This sleep deprivation has an impact on the addictive person's cognitive capacities such as memory and attention processing, decision making and fine motor coordination, and can contribute to cardiovascular and metabolic disorders.

Judith Grisel notes that alcohol acts like a "neurological sledgehammer", by acting throughout the brain to influence a multitude of brain circuits. Alcohol affects virtually all neural functioning including the shutdown of the brain's monitoring system resulting in the loss of inhibitions and the reduction of the normal constraints in the emotional region.

Substance abuse also contributes to what is called "alcohol myopia", a kind of "near-sightedness", or "tunnel vision". Substances like alcohol narrows the user's perceptual field resulting in a failure to consider alternatives; a failure to think through the negative and detrimental consequences of one's use; a failure to perspective-take and consider the impact of such usage on others, and on oneself.

Have you ever seen a horse pull a wagon wearing a set of blinders that limit its ability to look around and see alternative paths? Substance abuse, in its various different forms, can act in a similar manner, focusing an individual's attention on the immediate cravings, urges, emotional pain and the like. Substance use acts like a "channel selector" on a television set. This Patient Workbook is designed to help you choose different channels, remove your blinders.

> "I want, what I want, when I want it. I am a slave to my addiction."

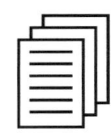

How did the brain become addicted, so this becomes the main channel, or message, that the brain sends? What can be done to change channels? The following points will help answer these questions.

1. Addictive behaviors affect the chemical and electrical *communication systems in the brain* in the form of blood flow, neurotransmitters and changes in receptor sites in the brain.

2. Addictive substances like alcohol, opioids, nicotine and other drugs activate (light up) the same brain circuits, as do behaviors linked to survival skills, eating, sex and the ability to bond with others.

3. The use of alcohol and drugs lead to a *surge* in a neurotransmitter called dopamine. Dopamine has been characterized as being the "wanting system" because it contributes to feelings of pleasure. The brain remembers this pleasure and wants it repeated. Substances can mimic and co-opt the dopamine system.

4. Moreover, research studies have demonstrated that just telling a person that his/her drink contains alcohol resulted in positive feelings of a "high', even if *no* alcohol was, in fact, included in the drink. Just the *expectation* of positive feelings is often sufficient to induce a "buzz" and accompanying substance abuse behaviors. Consistent with the previously noted observation that "Alcoholism is 10% drinking and 90% thinking", a person's expectation can play a critically inflated role in determining how he/she responds, especially in the presence of powerful triggers, cues and the social settings of how others are reacting.

   Not only do individuals learn to act at the psychological level in the *anticipation* of pleasure of ingesting various substances, but so does the brain. It is the *anticipation* of such pleasure, or what Judith Grisel describes as the "anxious lip-smacking foretaste of something of import that is just around the corner", that sets in motion the psychological arousal and craving to use substances that contribute to addiction.

5. The repetitive use of addictive substances induces the release of dopamine into various parts of the brain that impact the reward neural pathways that connect the upper part of the brain (frontal executive controlling lobes) with the lower emotional part of the brain (technically called the mesolimbic system consisting of the ventral tegmental and nucleus accumbens areas). The use of alcohol and drugs fool these areas with dopamine that can cause a reduction, and even a shutdown, to the neural reward system. The repeated use of substances *conditions* the brain to seek reinforcers at the expense of other neural pathways.

The use of substances become a *shortcut* way to the reward system. But in time the addict requires higher and higher doses, more and more of the substance intake, to achieve the same level of response ("buzz" or "high"). This increase in tolerance level leads to more drug-seeking behaviors, and to an increased level of cravings.

As a result, an "addiction trap" develops and the brain becomes more and more addicted. The dopamine "wanting system" makes one more susceptible to cues and reminders to use. The use of substances makes individuals more *cue sensitive*, even if they are *not* fully aware of this process.

"Remember the horse who wears blinders."

6. One of the things that make this "addiction cycle" worse is the experience of chronic stress and fatigue that results in increased cravings. (Remember that the use of substances "screws up" the sleep cycle). Chronic stress alters neurotransmitters of the brain that influence the capacity and tolerance to alcohol and drugs. As noted, chronic stress has a wear and tear impact on the body. Thus, a "loss spiral" develops.

7. The use of alcohol, especially in the form of binge drinking, contributes to impulsive disinhibiting behaviors. Binge drinking makes it easier for an addict's lower emotional brain to "hijack" the higher thinking brain's functioning. Under such influences, individuals are more likely to engage in "high-risk" behaviors such as drinking and driving, or shoplifting, aggressive behaviors, sexual acting out and the like.

Binge drinking is the consumption of five or more standard drinks in one sitting for men; for women, it is four or more drinks in one sitting, at least once in the previous thirty days. The differences between men and women is due to the fact that women metabolize alcohol differently than men.

Individuals who engage in binge drinking are *five times* more likely to have interpersonal problems in their relationships with their partner/spouse. The use of alcohol and substance abuse often precedes and co-occur with some form of domestic violence. Drug use, especially binging, *rewires* the brain's neural pathways so it thinks it needs more drugs. Cravings replace normal survival urges for sleep, sex and food. In order to fully recover, the adult brain needs to re-learn pre-drug use habits and develop new brain pathways. With consistent use of drugs, the brain establishes a new "normal". When drugs are not present, the resultant stress causes cravings that act as a potent drive and alters the motivational system.

Another major factor contributing to the addiction trap is the strong desire by addicts to avoid withdrawal symptoms and the unpleasant effects and accompanying physical symptoms. For example, protracted alcohol withdrawal is marked by feelings of nervousness, agitation, depression, loss of interest and sleep difficulties. These symptoms may persist for approximately three months during early remission.

Withdrawal is the result of *neuroadaptation* between the brain's development of *increased tolerance* to extended substance usage and the *rebound effect* due to the *removal of the drug*, establishing a new "set point". These two processes of tolerance and withdrawal occur simultaneously, in a dynamic manner. As addicts have reported:

> "I no longer use drugs to feel good. Instead, my alcohol and drug use serves to prevent my feeling sick. I do not feel 'normal' unless I am using my drug/alcohol."

There is a need to conduct a careful evaluation of withdrawal symptoms as part of any relapse prevention plan (see Module IX). This is especially true when the use of substances has become habitual, or on "autopilot"; that are elicited, or controlled by, cue-induced cravings (reminders to use). Such cues trigger surges in the dopamine brain neural circuitry that lead to "drug wanting" behaviors. Patients need to learn to cope with triggers. This is akin to training the brain to *unlearn associations*, or break the vicious cycle, between pre-potent cues and addictive behaviors; for example, using alcohol in the presence of a drinking buddy.

This takes effort, determination and patience. Brain recovery occurs during periods of sobriety, but *it takes time*. Brain dysfunction may exist for the first 6–18 months of sobriety. The most dramatic brain recovery from alcoholism is in the first three years of sobriety. The brain remains vulnerable, especially during the early stage of recovery.

With recovery and abstinence comes changes in both the structure and function of the brain, a form of "neurogenesis" and "neuroplasticity". There are changes in the brain's communication systems which include:

a) an increase in neurometabolites;

b) an increase in regional brain volume;

c) an increase in hippocampal volume resulting in improved short-term memory and long-term memory;

d) improved cognitive functioning and IQ improvement contributing to better social relationships.

Now that you have read (and hopefully, reread) the description of how the brain gets addicted, can you explain these processes to someone else? In your description can you describe the addiction trap? Can you include a description of how such factors as inheritance, exposure to early aversive childhood experiences, early usage, experience of ongoing chronic stress, social pressure and expectations, ready accessibility of substances, each contribute to an individual's vulnerability to become addicted and relapse?

In your description can you include an explanation of such terms as "alcohol myopia" (tunnel vision), cue sensitivity that triggers cravings, the dangers of binge drinking and altered tolerance levels? What about the avoidance of withdrawal symptoms in contributing to the "loss addictive spiral?"

Can you *now* describe what an individual has to do <u>to break the</u> vicious cycle *of addiction*? What are all the ways you can get out of, and avoid, the addiction trap, and begin to *reshape* your brain and behavior?

Here are a few points you can include in your explanation of how your brain gets addicted and, most importantly, contributes to an addiction trap.

1. People have different levels of vulnerability to begin with in becoming addicted to alcohol and to drugs. This is partly due to both what they inherited from their parents and what they experienced in their upbringing.

2. The abuse of alcohol and drugs changes the chemistry of the brain in terms of the communication network, called neurotransmitters.

3. In addition, the "emotional wanting" system of the brain can hijack the thinking part of the brain (frontal lobes), contribute to mood changes, sleep disturbance and behavior changes such as increased anger and aggression.

4. With continued use of alcohol and drugs, an individual can develop an increased tolerance which results in an addiction cycle, resulting in the need for more and more usage – a form of addiction trap.

5. The ongoing experience of chronic stress plus the development of mental disorders on top of substance abuse (a kind of "double whammy"), results in the wear and tear of the body and to the disruption of social relationships.

6. Finally, in an attempt to avoid the negative emotions and withdrawal symptoms, individuals' continued use results in their becoming more and more addicted, as a negative "loss spiral" develops. This spiral is exacerbated when there are cues and triggers to use present. Such cue sensitivity can exert an influence even when the individual is not fully aware of their presence. The urge or cravings to use may seem to appear "out of the blue." There is a need to develop and implement a Sobriety Script that

helps you look beyond any discomfort and cravings and keep in mind the longer-term benefits.

7. The brain is *not* a passive recipient to drug abuse, but the brain is *adaptive* in order to compensate for the changes associated with drugs. The brain is "clever" and automatically compensates for the impact of drugs. Drugs increase the rate of what is already going on in the brain, and in response produces a countervailing reaction. As the adage states, *"What goes up, must come down"*. This opponent process can lead to just the opposite set of emotional reactions. If the initial intake of the drug leads to a "high", then the more long-lasting eventual reaction will be a sustained "low". The positive initial feelings will gradually decrease over time. This eventually leads to the person getting little or no positive lasting feelings out of the drug. Instead, they experience the opposite discomforting negative feelings. In turn, individuals will need more and more of the drug to experience the same "high", as the brain develops tolerance to the drug.

Before we turn our attention to how you can break this vicious cycle, it is important to recognize the influence of the social context in influencing addictive behaviors. A good example is the follow up research on soldiers who served in Vietnam, where various forms of addictive drugs were readily available. Some 20% of these troops sought escape by taking narcotics. When they were followed up on their return to the States, only some 5% of the soldiers addicted in Vietnam evidenced drug abuse and relapse. This data highlights the power of social settings in influencing the use of substances.

WAYS TO BREAK THE ADDICTION TRAP

In order to break the vicious cycle and recondition one's brain, the *addict* and the *stressed-out* person has to *learn how to*:

1. Avoid and control cues ("reminders") that drive cravings;

2. Remove "blinders" and think through consequences, perspective-take and search for alternatives;

3. "Talk back" to the emotional part of your brain, and *not* allow it to hijack the thinking part of your brain;

4. Become aware of and tolerate and cope with withdrawal symptoms;

5. Be patient, but determined, and view any lapses as a "learning opportunity".

6. Develop and implement a Sobriety Script that helps you look beyond any discomfort and cravings and keep in mind the longer-term benefits.

EXERCISE 3
THE "BODY KEEPS SCORE" OF BOTH NEGATIVE AND POSITIVE EFFECTS: WAYS TO RESHAPE YOUR BRAIN

The previous sections indicate that the exposure to chronic stressors and the repetitive use of alcohol and drugs can have an impact on the brain that can cause cognitive and social deficits such as short-term memory loss, the loss of the ability to engage in abstract thinking and good decision making, and the loss of the ability to establish and maintain good social relationships with significant others in one's life. The ability to "bond" with your "frontal lobes" and with "trusted others" is *compromised* by the use of substances.

> The "body keeps score", as the psychiatrist Besell van der Kolk has observed.

HERE IS THE GOOD NEWS!

The body also keeps score of the impact of *positive emotions* and *resilient-engendering* behaviors. Remember that the brain is one of the most "plastic organs" in the body. Through two processes of "neuroplasticity" and "neurogenesis", you can *reshape your brain*, and begin your personal journey to abstinence and well-being. An example of the malleability of the brain is illustrated by the finding that when the area of the brain that processes visual stimuli is damaged, some of that area can be repurposed to enhance hearing. The brain has the ability to provide compensatory abilities.

> As noted, one's history is not one's destiny.

What this means is that when individuals engage in activities that elicit *positive emotions* such as optimism by maintaining a future hopeful orientation, forgiveness, gratitude, love and a sense of awe with nature and music, the brain responds in a regenerative manner. The brain has the ability to *compensate* and *repair* itself.

When individuals engage in an altruistic, helping fashion with others, by making a "gift" of one's experiences, and by engaging in "meaning-making" activities, individuals are not only helping others, but also "healing" their brains.

When brain researchers conduct neurological testing, using their PET scans and Functional Magnetic Resolutions equipment on individuals when they experience such positive emotions, various reward parts of their brain are activated.

Various synaptic plasticity (connections between neurons) are changed. Instead of turning to substances for a "high", "buzz", "avoidance of withdrawal symptoms" and the like, individuals who engage in resilience activities such as exercise, mindfulness and relaxation training, meditation and socially-engaging activities such as participating in recovery groups, have been found to improve their brain functioning and behavior.

Imagine a therapy that is readily available and could improve your cognitive functioning that had *no* bad side effects, and *cost nothing*. Such a Therapy has been known to writers, philosophers and lay people alike. What is this therapy? It is *interacting with nature*.

Research indicates that *nature heals* and improves cognitive functioning, reduces mental chatter and negative drug-seeking thinking, calms, reminds one of what is really important in life and enhances overall well-being.

Nature can be restorative. The experience of nature's sights, sounds, smells and even the "sounds of silence" can contribute to feelings of awe and the accompanying sense that one is part of humanity. Interacting with nature has been found to improve mood, increase attention and working memory capacity and increase well-being and mental and physical health.

Research indicates that there is a process called *epigenesis* that indicates that the social environment and resilient-engendering behaviors that elicit positive emotions can turn the genes in one's body on and off, and that these bodily benefits can be transmitted from one generation to another. For instance, if one has a high ACE score, one is not doomed. The brain is continually changing in response to your environment and your response. The individual's brain can become healthier through mindfulness practices, exercise, good nutrition, adequate sleep and healthy social relationships.

The remaining modules in this Patient Workbook will provide *specific practical* Exercises on ways you can increase positive emotions, improve social relationships and bolster your resilience.

You can also visit the Website roadmaptoresilience.wordpress.com to learn ways to bolster your resilience in six domains (physical, interpersonal, emotional, behavioral, cognitive and spiritual).

In summary, addictive disorders are complicated, but treatable. Knowing what predisposes an individual to develop and maintain addictive behaviors can be a protective device to add to your Coping Tool Box.

EXERCISE 4
UNDERSTANDING THE CONNECTION BETWEEN FEELINGS, THOUGHTS AND BEHAVIORS: USE OF A "CLOCK" METAPHOR

Here is a *simple* and *straight-forward* way for you to analyze any situation you encounter, so you can see how your feelings, thoughts, behaviors and the reactions of others are *interconnected*.

This analytic approach will provide a useful tool to break the vicious cycle and addictive trap.

For a moment, think of a Clock with a 12 o'clock, 3 o'clock, 6 o'clock and 9'o'clock.

12 o'clock will refer to any

- *external triggers* of what someone else does or says, or does not do or say, that elicits a response in you. It gets you going.
  It may include some *external cues*

- *internal triggers* that may reflect a memory, craving, urge, or sense of apprehension, or mood reminders

3 o'clock will refer to

- *primary feelings* that you experience immediately, at the time of the event such as feeling anxious, depressed, ashamed, lonely, and these emotions, in turn, may reflect and trigger "deep-seated" fears of rejection, abandonment and guilt.

- *secondary feelings* are experienced afterward, "down the road".

For instance, at the time when someone said something (12 o'clock), you may feel embarrassed or humiliated (*primary feelings*), but later on you may feel angry, or depressed (*secondary emotions*).

6 o'clock will refer to

- *your thinking processes*, automatic thoughts, your self-statements and images, your "internal dialogue" or what you tell yourself.

- it also refers to your appraisals, expectations, your attributions (causal explanations). For instance, your notion about whether the person did this "on purpose".

- it also refers to the deep-seated beliefs, attitudes and values you hold.

For instance, one may hold a set of beliefs that one is unlovable, or unworthy or that people *cannot* be trusted. Such beliefs color the way an individual views others, the future and what he/she says to oneself and feels.

9 o'clock will refer to

- *any specific behavior* you engage in, either by yourself or with others

- it also refers to how other people react and respond to whatever you did, or did not do.

In summary, Figure 2.1 illustrates this Clock metaphor. You can post this figure on your cell phone or on your computer as a screen saver.

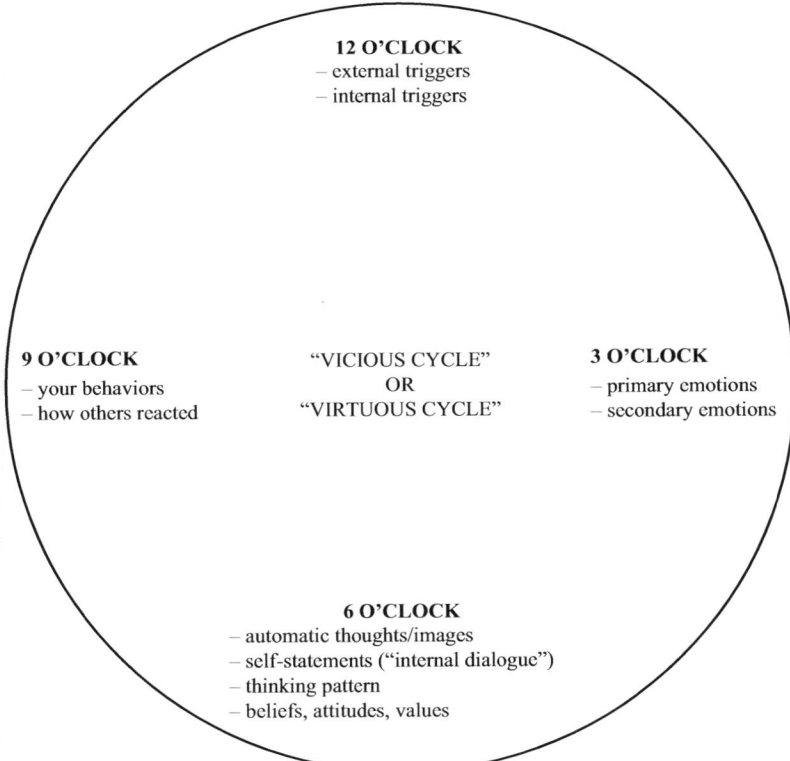

12 O'CLOCK
– external triggers
– internal triggers

9 O'CLOCK
– your behaviors
– how others reacted

"VICIOUS CYCLE"
OR
"VIRTUOUS CYCLE"

3 O'CLOCK
– primary emotions
– secondary emotions

6 O'CLOCK
– automatic thoughts/images
– self-statements ("internal dialogue")
– thinking pattern
– beliefs, attitudes, values

Figure 2.1

Now, let us consider the value of using the Clock analysis. You can take any situation you encounter, or any "story" someone else tells you, and you can ask the following questions:

12 o'clock

1. What happened? What was the trigger that set you off or got you going, or elicited some reaction?

2. Was the "trigger" something "external" that everyone could see?

3. Was the "trigger" something "internal" that emanated from you, within yourself?

3 o'clock

1. How did this make you feel *at the time* you were triggered? What were your immediate emotions? (Primary Emotions)

2. How did your emotions change over time? (Secondary Emotions)

   Note that both the primary and secondary emotions may be either negative or positive, or some combination of both sets of feelings.

3. One other set of questions concerning your 3 o'clock emotions: *What did you do with all of your feelings*? Did you stuff your feelings, or share your feelings with someone else, or try to drink your feelings away?

   For a moment, think about your feelings as a "commodity", or a "thing" you do something with.

4. Now ask yourself a *critical question*:

   What is the impact, what is the toll, what is the price you and others pay for the ways you handle your feelings?

   Is this the way you want things to be? How does handling your feelings in this manner help you achieve your treatment goals?

6 o'clock

1. What specific thoughts did you have *at the time* when this event occurred (12 o'clock), and when you had specific emotional reactions (3 o'clock)?

2. What did you "tell yourself" at the time and what *lingered* afterwards?

3. Did any specific expectations, appraisals and beliefs get triggered by this situation that, in turn, further impacted your feelings?

4. How did your thoughts and feelings influence what you did; how you behaved and interacted with others? (9 o'clock)

9 o'clock

1. Given the way you view events (12 o'clock), and how you feel about them (3 o'clock), and what thoughts you had at the time and down the road (6 o'clock), what did *you do* and *how did others respond* (9 o'clock)?

With the assistance of a Treatment Team, they can help you learn to analyze any situation, even when you are tempted to use substances, or when you are feeling stressed-out into these *four components.*

There is *no* situation that you cannot break down into

12 o'clock – triggers

3 o'clock – feelings

6 o'clock – thoughts

9 o'clock – behaviors and reactions of others.

Note that sometimes you can begin the analysis with your feelings (3 o'clock), and then see what accompanying behaviors you engage in (9 o'clock), and then figure out what thoughts you had (6 o'clock).

You can go around the clock in *any direction.* The goal is to better understand that you are *not* a *mere "victim"* of a situation, nor a victim of your feelings, urges, thoughts and the like.

You can break any vicious cycle. The remaining modules in this Patient Workbook will teach you ways to break this vicious cycle that contributes to an addiction trap.

One last observation, you can use the Clock analysis to develop a "virtuous cycle". If something goes well, such as you used your refusal skills, or your mindfulness skills, to cope with a temptation to use, you can ask yourself the following questions:

12 o'clock

1. What just happened? What was the potential temptation that I handled?

3 o'clock

1. How did that make me feel? (For example, proud, more self-confident)

2. What did I do with these feelings? (Did I share them with anyone else? Did I pat myself on the back for how I handled the temptation? Did I record these events and feelings in my journal?)

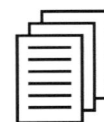

6 o'clock

1. What did I tell myself that bolsters my sense of confidence and hope? What post event analysis can I replay in my mind's eye, as a form of mental rehearsal for handling future such temptations?

9 o'clock

1. How did others respond to what I did, or did *not* respond?

2. Can I do this again, so I can experience a virtuous cycle?

How can you turn the vicious cycles in your life into virtuous cycles? You can break the cycle at any point.

DISCUSSION STARTERS FOR MODULE II

"Feelings listened to and being understood can rewire the brain."

"Alcohol makes you feel like you're supposed to feel when you're not drinking."

"The brain is the most plastic (changeable) organ in the body."

"The body keeps score not only of the impact of trauma, but also of resilience. Positive emotions can change the structure and function of the brain."

RECOVERY VOICE II: GROUP TREATMENT AND GROUP HUGS

> Group therapy is the most common form of treatment for individuals with various forms of substance abuse and co-occurring disorders in both inpatient and outpatient centers.
>
> The degree of group cohesion is the most critical feature contributing to lasting changes.

The most valuable part of my treatment were the group meetings with my fellow patients. I came to realize that I was not alone in struggling with my addiction problems. I was no longer isolated.

Our therapist was masterful in establishing and maintaining rapport and group cohesion. Over the course of our sessions, I came to see that the group members language shifted from "I" and "You" to "We".

Our group therapist did three things that really worked. First, she would invite a different member of the group to act as a "co-therapist" each session. The assigned patient was asked to keep notes during the session, and at the end of the meeting to provide the group a summary of the main points, and ask for group feedback. Members were asked to make a "commitment" of what they will work on before the next meeting.

Second, she would begin each session with a Discussion Starter taken from this Patient Workbook. The group members are invited to discuss their understanding of this Quote. My two favorite Discussion Starters are:

"There is no situation so bad that by your own efforts you cannot make it worse."

"If you have skeletons in your closet, you had best teach them how to dance."

These discussions set the tone and subsequent theme for each session. Patients were invited to bring in their own Quote to be discussed. The patient had to explain to the group why he or she chose that Quote.

Finally, where I learned the most was how she used the Clock metaphor on a group basis. She put on the wall a poster with the 12, 3, 6 and 9 o'clock reminders. She would go around the room and ask the various group members a series of questions to identify "triggers" that led them to use substances.

- "What was your trigger that got you going?"

- "What set you off?"

- "How did that event increase your urge to use?"

She even got somewhat reticent patients to provide examples of what they experienced. She was a master using the "art of questioning" asking mainly

"What" and "How" questions and a guided discovery approach. (I am telling you that I do not think Socrates could have done a better job.)

She would then ask the group members:

"What, if anything, did these various triggers have in common?"

This naturally led to a discussion of the 3 o'clock analysis of the feelings they had in the situations.

"When that happened (triggering events), how did you feel at the time?"

"Have others of you had similar feelings?

"What do these feelings have in common?"

Once she elicited these feelings, and what feelings still linger she would ask group members:

"What did you do with all of your feelings?"

She would have the patients come to view their feelings as a kind of "commodity" that they did something with. The group members would often say that they "stuffed their feelings", or that they "drank their feelings away", or that they "engaged in some high risky behavior". She would then go onto asking the key question:

"If you do that with your feelings, then what is the impact, what is the toll, what is the price you and others are paying? And, is that the way you want it to be?"

Even if some patients would say, "I don't know", she would say "I don't know either. How can *we* go about finding out?" She was an expert at using her befuddlement and bemusement, as a way of engaging patients in coming up with suggestions.

(I tell you if they ever make re-runs of the television detective program Columbo with Peter Falk, I would nominate our therapist to play the part.)

Next, she would tackle the 6 o'clock thinking processes, by asking about what automatic thoughts (inner speech), they had at the time of the triggering event and what still lingers now. She would highlight how the individuals' thinking processes and Mindset played a role in how they responded.

Finally, she would go around the room soliciting what people did or did not do, and how others responded. She helped the participants to appreciate the interconnections between their feelings, thoughts and behaviors and how they inadvertently, unwittingly and perhaps even unknowingly play a critical role in creating a vicious cycle. If this is actually occurring, then what could the patients do about it?

It was *not* too big of a step, for someone to say that they should *break the vicious cycle.* She would ask, *"How are you now going about 'breaking your Vicious Cycle'? Are there better ways to break the cycle, besides using some form of substances?"*

The focus of the group discussions and practice sessions was to develop better and healthier ways to break the vicious cycle.

Each session ended with a group hug.

I gave this description to my group therapist to see if I had captured what she does. She gave me permission to include this description in this Patient Workbook.

MODULE III

Collaborative Goal-Setting

Ways to Nurture Hope

Exercise 1: SMART Goals: What They Are and How to Use Them

Exercise 2: How Good Are You in Giving Advice?

Exercise 3: Putting Together My Goal Sheet

Exercise 4: Goal-Setting for Habit Change

Exercise 5: How Would I Know If My Goal-Setting Worked?

Exercise 6: Future Imagery Planning

Exercise 7: A Barriers Analysis: Possible Reasons Why I Won't Change

See Appendix A for a discussion of what treatments "work" for individuals with addiction and co-occurring disorders.

One way to *nurture hope* is to develop and work toward achieving meaningful, attainable goals. As a result of working on this Module, you will be able to achieve the following:

1. Develop SMART goals, in collaboration with your Treatment Team that nurtures hope;

2. Explain to someone what is involved in implementing SMART goals and describe how you can use these steps when working on your treatment goals;

3. Offer the *reasons* why you are trying to change, as well as the *reasons* ("excuses") why individuals fail to achieve their goals;

4. Write out a specific treatment Action Plan on ways you can monitor your progress, and learn how to "take credit" for the changes you have accomplished;

5. Learn how to anticipate and handle any potential barriers or obstacles that may arise.

EXERCISE 1
SMART GOALS: WHAT THEY ARE AND HOW TO USE THEM

To be successful one needs to have SMART goals. A goal is something I want to get, or something I want to have happen, *and* I am *willing to work for it*.

What are SMART goals and why are they important?

Your Goals Must Be Specific

"I will do X in situation Y and observe the following changes."

Vague and abstract goals are unlikely to be attainable.

Your Goals Must Be *Measurable*

"You and others must be able to observe your progress relative to where you began, or what you are doing or not doing now (your baseline behavior). You need to be able to measure or count your behaviors in some way and track your progress on a regular basis."

Your Goals Must Be *Achievable*

"Your goals need to be doable and within your capability to 'perform'" (Not too easy and not too hard)."

Your Goals Must Be *Relevant* and *Realistic*

"This means that your treatment goals must be something that you and others really want."

Your Goals Must Be *Time-Limited*

"This means you need to have both short-term, intermediate and long-term goals."

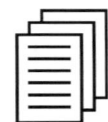

In summary,

S – Specific

M – Measurable

A – Achievable

R – Relevant and Realistic

T – Time-limited

MY PERSONAL ACTION PLAN: HOW TO APPLY MY SMART GOALS

1. Develop an Action Plan of targeted goals of what you wish to achieve. Your stated goals should answer the following questions: "What, when, where, how often and with whom" should I try these behaviors?

2. Prioritize your goals. What sub-goals should come first before the final goal is possible? Remember, "Think big, but Act small". Every big goal is accomplished in smaller *doable* steps. Start off with goals that are most achievable, so you have the best chance to succeed.

   Set goals that are important and relevant to your life, really meaningful and consistent with your values. Values can orient you toward your goals. Focus your attention on a few important goals. Keep it simple!

3. What immediate one or two things should you do to get stated? For example,

   "If this were a friend's goal, what advice would you offer so he/she can get started?"

4. Make sure that the goals you choose are doable. Start small and then make your goals gradually more challenging, as compared to setting unrealistic goals. Focus on initiating or starting *new behaviors*, rather than on trying to eliminate negative behaviors. Frame your goals in "positive terms". For example, instead of having the goal of "not shouting" set the goal of "speaking calmly".

   Remind yourself that "small steps can lead to big changes". It is like throwing a small stone into a pond and watching how a small splash can generate ripples that have an expanding effect.

   "Is there some way to moderate my use of substances and reduce the harm to myself?"

   "What is one thing, even if it is a little thing, which I can accomplish today that will help me move in the direction I want to go?"

   For some individuals their treatment goal is designed Harm Reduction which is to reduce the harm associated with using drugs and other risky behaviors without requiring abstinence. The goal is to bring about positive change toward risk. Harm Reduction is designed to mitigate harm and help individuals take ownership by means of stable moderation. For some individuals such Harm Reduction is the first step toward abstinence. It is critical for therapists to meet their clients "where they are at" and collaborate on the treatment goals.

5. What would be the *first signs* that you are making progress? What small steps would indicate that you are inching toward your goal? Who would *notice your changes*? What would they see changed? How will these changes make you feel and indicate that you are on the right track?

6. Use Solution Talk that focuses on the language of what works, rather than on the language of what is wrong. Solution Talk puts the spotlight on discovering and implementing solutions in the here and now with the goal of improving the future. Solution Talk includes "How" and "What" questions. For example:

    "How would I like things to be?"

    "How have I handled problems/challenges like this in the past?"

    "How did I do that?"

    "How can I use my coping skills and resources in this situation?"

    "What can I do differently?"

    "What is working? Can I do more of this?"

    "What is a first step that I can take?"

7. Be optimistic, but do not overshoot your goals. Anticipate possible barriers and consider what you will do if you encounter roadblocks or obstacles. Develop back-up plans and proactive skills to address "Whenever" and "If then" statements:

    "Whenever I encounter ... I will ..."

    "If ... then" plans.

    Don't be a perfectionist. Learn from setbacks. View any lapses as a "learning opportunity", rather than as an occasion to "catastrophize".

8. Is there a way to involve significant others in your Action Plan?

9. You should have an end point in mind in order to keep you motivated. Set a *realistic deadline* and *doable time frame* for achieving your short-term, intermediate and long-term goals. "What are your goals behind your goals? How will achieving your treatment goals improve your quality of life?"

10. Write down and share with others the reasons why you wish to work on these goals. Offer explanations to yourself and to others why you are engaged in these activities.

11. Who can you *share* these goal plans with? Make a *public commitment* of what you are doing with significant others whom you care about. What would you like them to say or do that would increase the likelihood that you can achieve your treatment goals? What can you say or do that can help them be of assistance such as help you avoid temptations, help with triggers that contribute to lapses, and the like? How can you approach and engage significant others to assist and support your Action Plan?

12. *Anticipate possible barriers* and have a plan and back-up strategies to deal with any individual and external barriers/obstacles that may get in the way of your goal-directed behavior. Prepare ahead of time for any potential barriers and develop back-up plans that you can practice ahead of time.

13. Monitor your progress and reinforce yourself for your effort and strategy use, not only for your outcomes. Take credit for your efforts and for trying. See the connections between your efforts and the results. Consider the ways you "planned, noticed, caught yourself, avoided high risk situations, distracted yourself, reframed the temptations, did 'urge surfing' and the like". Keep a diary of the risk situations and what you did to handle these, like lower your cue sensitivity to use substances.

14. Choose what are called Mastery Goals versus Performance Goals. Mastery Goals are established by yourself and reflect intrinsic motivation that comes from personal desires. When your treatment goals originate from you, you are more likely to demonstrate persistence, grit and determination and accept any mistakes or lapses as part of learning. You are more likely to demonstrate curiosity and "play detective" in figuring out what went wrong and what can be done next time.

In contrast, Performance Goals are established and evaluated by others. Such imposed goals by others are more likely to lead to giving up, fear of failure and lead to lower motivation and drive to achieve.

What type of treatment goals have you set for yourself and how many of these steps have you included?

Now, let's see how you can use all of this information in doing the next set of Exercises.

EXERCISE 2
HOW GOOD ARE YOU IN GIVING ADVICE?

Imagine that a friend or relative came to you and said:

> "I have difficulty following through on my New Year's Eve Resolutions, or on my plans to change a behavior that I need to alter."

What specific advice could you give on what he/she needs to do to increase the likelihood that he/she could be successful?

In your own words describe how he/she can set up SMART goals.

EXERCISE 3
PUTTING TOGETHER MY GOAL SHEET

MY GOAL SHEET

A goal is something I want to get or something I want to have happen and I am *willing to work for it*.

My goal is (be specific):

The changes I want to make are:

The most important reasons for changing are:

The specific steps I plan to take in changing are/or the advice I would give someone else to achieve this goal is:

How can I get started? What *small changes* can I make to begin with?

The ways other people can help me are:

Person

Possible ways they can help

I will know if my plan is working if:

Who else would notice the changes? What would he/she observe?

Some things that could interfere with my plans are … and some possible solutions are …

If my Action Plan does *not* work, I will use my back-up plan ("I will be on the lookout for …"; "Whenever I see/hear … I will do …"; "I will tell myself …";

"I will ask for help from …").

The benefits to me and others from changing are …

Someone I can share my Personal Goal with is …

Some specific things I can do to bring about these changes are: (Next to each specific action you can do to change indicate an 0% to 100% level of confidence that you will be able to do each activity – 100% is completely confident).

What I can do is:

1. _____ % confident

2. _____ % confident

3. _____ % confident

I can see how my efforts made a difference ("take credit" for change). Give examples:
I can reinforce myself, pat myself on the back, share my positive feeling with … about my efforts. I can do a virtuous cycle Clock analysis of what I did and how it made me feel.

EXERCISE 4
GOAL-SETTING FOR HABIT CHANGE

Give an example of an unwanted deeply ingrained overlearned habit you want to change.

How does your unwanted habit affect you?

How does your unwanted habit affect others in your life?

Write down the *reasons* that this concerns you. Why do you want to change this unwanted habit?

How can you use your SMART goals to change this habit?

Keep in mind, the author Mark Twain's adage:

"Habit is habit and not to be flung out the window by any man, but coaxed downstairs one step at a time."

EXERCISE 5
HOW WOULD I KNOW IF MY GOAL-SETTING WORKED?

This exercise is designed to help you *evaluate* if the treatment goals you set did work. You can use a procedure called Goal Attainment Scaling, whereby you identify for specific targeted behaviors what would constitute 100% improvement in that area, 50% improvement and 0% improvement. You can *now* compare your present level of improvement against what you had identified as what would constitute *significant improvement*.

What will it take to improve further? What is getting in the way and how can this be addressed?

List two or three treatment goals you have identified. Now indicate for each treatment goal specific ways you would like your behavior to change. Indicate what a 100% improvement would look like? What would 50% change look like? What would 0% change look like? What would each level of behavioral improvement look like?

SPECIFIC WAYS YOUR BEHAVIOR SHOULD CHANGE

	Minimal Improvement	Moderate Improvement	Significant Improvement
	0% Change	50% Change	100% Change
Target Behavior 1			
Target Behavior 2			
Target Behavior 3			

EXERCISE 6
FUTURE IMAGERY PLANNING

Consider the following advice offered by the famous golfer Jack Nicklaus. He stated:

Before every shot, I go to the movies inside my head. Here is what I see. First, I see the ball where I want it to finish, nice and white and sitting up high on the bright green grass. Then I see the ball going there, its path and trajectory, and its behavior on landing. The next scene shows me making the kind of swing that will turn the previous images into reality. These home movies are a key to my concentration and to my positive approach to every shot.

Note that in this example, Nicklaus was able to *work backwards* from his goal and then picture in his mind's eye the steps involved in achieving each sub-goal.

Select a treatment goal you wish to achieve, the end-state and work backwards, and envision, using imagery, how you can achieve each sub-goal. After playing this scenario out in your mind's eye, now write out these various sub-goals.

EXERCISE 7
A BARRIERS ANALYSIS: POSSIBLE REASONS WHY I WON'T CHANGE

Take a moment to write down a health-related behavior you think you should be engaging in.

For example,

"I should exercise more";

"I should lose weight";

"I should go for a colonoscopy";

"I should drink less."

Health-related behavior I should change.

Now, be honest with yourself and write down *all of the reasons* you do *not* engage in this health-related activity.

Compare your reasons you do *not* change with the following categories of reasons. There are *three* major classes of reasons ("excuses") why folks do not change their health-related behaviors. How many of these reasons did you offer?

CLASSES OF REASONS: HOW PEOPLE CONVINCE THEMSELVES AND OTHERS NOT TO CHANGE THEIR HEALTH-RELATED BEHAVIORS

1. People may act like "Doubting Thomases" and questioning scientists. They question the validity or usefulness of engaging in the specific health-related behaviors. For example:

"It won't work for me."

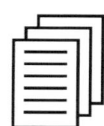

"I have seen other people engage in these behaviors (keep smoking, drinking) and they live long, productive lives."

"I read about folks who exercise and jog and they had a heart attack and died."

2. People may act like economists and they weigh the benefits and costs, the pros and cons of changing. They focus on potential barriers and obstacles such as the time involved, expense, possible side-effects and social pressure for not changing their behavior. As a result, they procrastinate and end up *not* doing anything.

"I am telling you the side-effects are worse than what I now experience."

"If I give up smoking, I will gain weight and die. Choose your poison."

"If I don't drink, I won't be able to sleep/cope, be as creative, and I will lose my friends and be rejected."

3. People may hold *deep-seated beliefs* that lead them to refrain from engaging in health-related behaviors. Some beliefs may be shared by their group or culture that they are part of. These beliefs may include:

"We are all going to die of something, why change?" (Fatalistic beliefs)

"I don't like anyone telling me how to live my life. I want to be in control.'

"I am beyond help and I lack the necessary willpower to succeed."

Now go back to your list of reasons that you wrote down. Did you act like:

- A "Doubting Thomas" questioning scientist

- An excuse-making economist

- A committed belief-holder who refutes the need to change?

What would it take for you to change? See Appendix B on steps to enhance your motivation to change.

What are your reasons to change?

SUMMARY

SELF-CHECKLIST OF HOW YOU CAN CREATE AN ACTION PLAN TO ACHIEVE YOUR TREATMENT GOALS

As you create your Action Plan, here are some questions to ask yourself.

1. Is the specific goal that I intend to work on include identifiable behavioral terms? (The "what, when, how, with whom")

2. What is the expected time period to achieve this goal?

3. Are there sub-goals that need to be accomplished first in my Action Plan?

4. What are the specific skills and supports that I will need to achieve this goal?

5. On a 0% to 100% scale, how confident am I that I can achieve this goal?

6. Have I told anyone and shared my goal or plans, and engaged them in my goal-setting process (made a public commitment)? How can others in my life help me achieve my treatment goals? What have I done to enlist their support?

7. Can I anticipate any possible barriers and obstacles that might get in the way of achieving my goals? How can I learn to anticipate and handle these possible obstacles? What are my back-up plans if my original Action Plan does not work?

8. How will I, and others, observe any changes in order to tell if I am making progress?

9. How can I reinforce myself and take credit for the changes I have been instrumental in bringing about?

10. Why should I go through this entire process of goal-setting? What reasons can I offer myself and others for working on these goals? When I achieve my goals how will that make me feel? How will my life be different if I achieve my objectives? What is the value of doing all this work? I can keep a diary of both my efforts and outcomes.

Asking yourself these questions on a *regular basis* will be helpful in you achieving your treatment goals. These questions are putting the frontal lobe of your brain in charge, so that your behavior is not "hijacked" by your cravings, urges, temptations and the lower emotional part of your brain. You have choices.

DISCUSSION STARTERS FOR MODULE III

"History is not destiny."

"The past is never dead. It's not even past" (William Faulkner) (It is part of us and determines how we approach the present and future).

"History, despite its wrenching pain cannot be unlived, but if faced with courage need not be lived again." (Maya Angelou, "On the pulse of morning")

"Setting SMART goals nurtures hope."

"Short sightedness is ingrained in human nature. We need an optimist's telescope."

RECOVERY VOICE III: THE ROLE OF THE THERAPEUTIC ALLIANCE

> It matters not only what treatment is being offered, but who offers it.

My therapist kept asking me the same question over and over:

"Do you ever find yourself, out there, in your daily life, asking yourself the type of questions that we ask each other right here in therapy?"

After a while, I came to recognize that I had actually taken my therapist's voice with me. I had become my own therapist and my own "emotional detective". I have had other therapists in the past, but this therapist was different. He was able to create a collaborative working alliance and asked my feedback on a session-by-session basis. Here are some of the things he did that made a difference in my life.

He was non-judgemental, caring, compassionate, supportive, kind, and I felt respected, safe and heard.

He was collaborative in setting my treatment goals. I had a "love affair" with my drugs and I didn't want to give them up. So we set up a Harm Reduction program for my use, so I wouldn't harm myself.

He nurtured hope as we worked together in setting up an agreed set of treatment goals and the ways to achieve them. He offered me hope, looking for small successes. He evoked my Change Talk and he highlighted the language of possibilities.

Even when I lapsed and started to use drugs again, I remembered him saying, "I will work with you until we find what works for you. We can figure out what are all of the barriers and address each one at a time."

I told him I wasn't going to give up my coping behavior of using drugs until I have better ways to replace them. We worked on the "emotional pain" that was behind my use.

When I missed an appointment, my therapist sent me a text to see if I was okay. He conveyed a sense of trust and confidence in me, even when I was still engaging in risky drug behaviors. I worked hard to make him proud of me.

He showed great empathy and was sensitive and understanding of my feelings and struggles. He listened attentively and reflected what I said, moving me along toward recovery. He helped me consider ways to break my cycle of addiction.

He would say, "My job is to put myself out of business with you and have you become your own therapist." I am working on this transition.

Ways to Strengthen Your Emotional Coping Tool Box

Exercise 1: The Nature and Impact of Negative Emotions

Exercise 2: Ways to Self-Regulate Negative Emotions

Exercise 3: Ways to Self-Soothe, Tolerate and Accept Your Negative Emotions

Exercise 4: Ways to Increase Your Positive Emotions

Your Treatment Team Can Help You Learn and Practice These Coping Skills.

Sometimes the triggers for drinking and using substances, or for experiencing stress, are external events like exposure to cues ("reminders") to which individuals are remarkably sensitive. Another external trigger may be the *behaviors of others* such as social pressure to drink or use drugs, or interpersonal conflict with others. These triggers are referred to as (12 o'clock) *external triggers* that can elicit urges and cravings and can set you off, and put you on a path of lapses, and perhaps toward a total relapse.

This module will highlight how *internal triggers*, an individual's feelings, mood and cravings can be the catalyst for lapses or slips (3 o'clock).

A second source of internal triggers are thinking processes, beliefs and 'stories" that individuals tell themselves and others (6 o'clock). The role that your thinking processes play will be considered in the next module, V.

The Exercises in both Modules IV and V are designed to help you *increase your awareness* of internal triggers and *strengthen* your Coping Tool Box.

In this module,

Exercise 1 begins with a consideration of the nature and function of *negative emotions* that can undermine your personal journey of recovery and well-being.

Exercise 2 will provide examples of specific ways you can *self-regulate* negative emotions.

Exercise 3 will provide examples of ways to *self-soothe*, *tolerate* and *accept* your negative emotions.

Exercise 4 will consider ways to increase your *positive emotions* using a variety of coping tools such as *exercise*, mindfulness and relaxation activities, *engaging* in a "bucket list" of *pleasant activities*, and employing supportive *social relationships*.

Recall from Module III on psycho-education, the interconnectedness between one's feelings, thoughts, behaviors and resultant consequences that can create a *vicious cycle* and a "loss spiral" that contributes to relapse. This module on emotions will help you learn ways to *break* the <u>vicious cycle</u>, and develop a positive *virtuous cycle* of resilience and well-being.

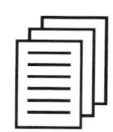

EXERCISE 1
THE NATURE AND IMPACT OF NEGATIVE EMOTIONS

Feelings and thoughts are two sides of the same coin. What and how you think can influence how you feel and behave. But, our feelings can, in turn, influence how you think and behave. Feelings can act like a television remote channel selector. If you are depressed, then you are likely to retrieve or call up other depressive memories. If you experience physiological cravings and urges, they may act like "commandments" to use substances. Your feelings, cravings, thoughts and behaviors can snowball leading you to operate on an "autopilot" habitual mode of substance use.

How can you break this *vicious* and self-destructive cycle? A good place to start is to increase your knowledge and awareness about the nature and impact of emotions. Here are some facts to keep in mind.

SOME FACTS ABOUT EMOTIONS

1. Emotions are sources of information; a signal worth listening to.

2. Negative and positive emotions often *coexist*. It is not an either-or situation.

3. Individuals are *not* mere victims of one's feelings (and one's thoughts) and you can learn to regulate, tolerate and accept your feelings.

4. There is *nothing wrong* with experiencing negative emotions such as anxiety, depression, guilt, shame, anger, grief and the like. It is what one does with these feelings and states that is critical.

5. No feeling lasts forever. Both the body, and in particular the brain, have the ability to adapt to emotional changes and drug ingestion. For example, the body has various mechanisms to maintain "set points" of body temperature at 98.6 °F. If the body's temperature is too high or too low, the body calls into play the mechanisms of sweating and shivering, accordingly. In the same way, if your emotions become too negative or too positive in intensity and frequency, the brain has the ability to engage in what are called a set of "opponent processes" to maintain an emotional "set point". This mechanism known as "emotional homeostasis" helps individuals establish and maintain a rebound stability.

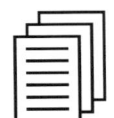

As described in Exercise 2, individuals can choose to engage in behaviors that elicit opposite emotional reactions. The concept of Instead behaviors can be used to reduce cravings and stave off withdrawal symptoms. The use of drugs influences these emotional set points, but they are reversible.

6. Finally, for a moment, think of your feelings as a "commodity" that you do something with. What do you do with your intense negative emotions? For example, some people report that they:

"Stuff their feelings."

"Drink my feelings away."

"Avoid experiencing my emotions. Suppress them and keep them under wraps."

"Not share my feelings with others."

If individuals do these things with their feelings, then what are the *impact*, *toll and price* that they and others are going to pay? How one copes with negative feelings has both a physical and social impact on themselves and on others in their lives.

For example, intense negative emotions can *hijack* the self-controlling, executive portion of your brain and compromise the neurotransmitter communication system between the upper part of your brain (frontal lobe area) from the lower emotional part of your brain (subcortical area such as the amygdala).

Negative emotions, especially if prolonged over time, can contribute to a compromised immune system that increases the likelihood of a number of physical illnesses (hypertension, cardiovascular disease and others).

The experience of chronic stress that piles up over time, and the accompanying negative emotions, affect not only the structure and function of the brain, but they can increase stress hormones (like cortisol) that prevent troubling memories from fading. Cumulative stress responses and excessive negative feelings can make you more sensitive and responsive to cues and reminders to use again.

For example, individuals often continue to drink and use drugs because they want to avoid the negative emotional and physical symptoms of withdrawal systems. In this way they are self-medicating. They use again in order to relax, sleep, socialize and cope.

Please give an example of when your negative feelings and your emotions have:

"hijacked, overwhelmed, ramped up, magnified your fears, shortened your fuse, shut down the executive thinking part of your brain"

Give an example of when you time-slided back to your habitual ways of coping (autopilot automatic, impulsive style of thinking). For example, some people engage in "high-risk" adrenaline-rush behaviors in order to avoid and combat negative emotions. What are alternative, more constructive ways to cope with your negative emotions?

EXERCISE 2
WAYS TO SELF-REGULATE
NEGATIVE EMOTIONS

Let's begin with the *good news*. You can learn how to regulate, control, tolerate, blunt, label and tame your emotions, surmount your fears, orchestrate, accept and share your feelings. You can also *reshape* your brain and learn how to "talk back" to the emotional part of your brain (the emotional alarm system – the amygdala).

Here is a "game plan" on ways to begin the healing and coping processes.

1. Become an "emotional detective" in learning how to *notice early warning signs* of the onset of negative emotions, bodily cravings and urges to use, and the onset of emotional distress.

2. Be aware of the high-risk settings and cues, and emotional "red flags" that can elicit a negative mood.

3. Label or name and then tame your emotions. You can rate the intensity of your emotions on a 0% to 100% scale of Subjective Units of Distress (SUDs), where 100% is the "worst" level of distress you have ever experienced and 0% is minimally disturbed in terms of your emotional distress.

   You can keep track and record your SUDs score in your Workbook. You will be able to do a Clock analysis of this episode as shown below.

   What Happened:

   12 o'clock – What was the trigger? (external or internal or both)

   3 o'clock – How did that make me feel? Now give a SUDs rating.

   6 o'clock – What did I tell myself? What were my thoughts?

   9 o'clock – What did I do, or *not* do? How did others react?

How Good of an Emotional Detective Can You Become?

4. Engage in *opposite behaviors* to your negative emotions. Incorporate and make prominent in your self-talk the word "instead". Look beyond your current negative emotions.

"Instead of keeping my feelings a secret and stuffing them, I am going to share them with a supportive trusting other."

"Instead of letting my emotions take over, I am going to take a Time Out and use my thinking skills."

"Instead of avoiding situations and magnifying my fears, I can be courageous and confront these situations, with the help of others."

"Instead of giving into my negative emotions and cravings, I can talk back to my amygdala (emotional alarm system)."

"Instead of managing my overwhelming feelings with drugs, I can quit and be kinder to my 'inner voice'."

"Instead of coping with my symptoms of trauma with substances, I can work with my therapist about the emotional pain behind my drug use."

"Instead of having harmful addictions, I can develop and engage in positive addictions (like exercise, gardening, hobbies, enjoy nature)."

"Instead of getting all up tight and tense, I can relax – use tactical breathing."

"Instead of dwelling on the past and ruminating, I can engage in mindfulness, focusing on the present."

"Instead of drinking my bad feelings away, I can ask for help from someone I trust."

"Instead of attacking someone because of my anger, I can take a Time Out and talk about it later when I cool down and take a Time In."

"Instead of trying to control my emotions, I can learn to accept them."

"I can learn to change my feelings by acting opposite to my current emotions. I can learn that I can feel good and I can make it so."

Count the Number of Times You Use the Word "Instead" when Talking to Others, as Well as when Talking to Yoursel.

5 Helpful Thoughts that "I Can Tell My Brain" in Order to Cope with My Cravings and Negative Emotions:

"I have resisted my cravings before and I can do it again."

"My cravings in the past have passed and these will too."

"I can delay/procrastinate my cravings. Delay is better than just giving in."

"I have used my drinking/drugs to calm down (self-medicate, avoid withdrawal symptoms), as a 'crutch' in the past. Now, I can use my drug-free relaxation/mindfulness coping skills."

"I can use my future imagery planning like Jack Nicklaus."

"I have to think through the drink (drug use) and remind myself (image in detail) the bad things that can happen to me and the people I care for."

"If one coping strategy does not work, try something else, but the important thing is to keep working on it."

"Never give up. A slip does not have to become a relapse."

"I have the grit and courage to stay clean."

"I now have multiple ways to bring joy to what was my joyless life."

"I can down-regulate my (urges, negative emotions, withdrawal symptoms)."

In summary, in order to regulate your negative feelings, you can:

1. Increase awareness and become an "emotional detective".

2. Be on the lookout for early warning signs.

3. Label, tame and rate the level of emotionality – Use SUDs: 0%–100%).

4. Conduct a Clock analysis.

5. Engage in opposite behaviors: Instead

6. Use *relaxation skills* and *tactical breathing*.

Tactical breathing involves learning how to use slow diaphragmatic breathing. Take a moment to conduct a "body scan". Ask yourself, "How do I feel in my body?" Use your body as a clue to find out how you are feeling. Now focus on your breathing.

1. Breathe in slowly for six counts through your nose.

2. Hold for two counts.

3. Breathe out for 10 seconds through your mouth.

4. Hold for two counts.

5. Repeat.

Feel free to alternate breathing in and out that best suits you. The breath in count should be shorter than the breath out count.

The goal of tactical breathing is to learn to take normal breaths and to extend the process of exhaling in order to enhance relaxation. By using tactical breathing, you can lower your heart rate by 6 to 10 beats per minute and, in turn, lower your overall arousal level.

Another way to relax is to use "safe place imagery" that is calming. Focus your mind on this image.

"Talk back" to my Amygdala – change my "self-talk".

Use tactical breathing and positive calming imagery.

Remember, like any skill, in order to master these coping procedures so they become automatic requires *deliberate practice*. Not just any type of practice, but practice that has specific SMART goals in mind.

You have to be able to tell others the *reasons* why using these coping tools are needed and how they will work. What might get in the way? How will you handle any potential obstacles/barriers? How much confidence do you have in using each skill?

EXERCISE 3
WAYS TO SELF-SOOTHE, TOLERATE AND ACCEPT YOUR NEGATIVE EMOTIONS

The mind loves to hang around in the past and become preoccupied with the uncertainty of the future. Both of these highly-charged activities can elicit negative emotions. This exercise will provide ways to *stay in the present* using *mindfulness* and *acceptance* activities. A number of self-soothing activities are listed and you can choose from this list. Which of these activities have you used in the past? Are there any of these activities that you could consider adding to your coping repertoire?

Mindfulness is a set of skills, involving ongoing, moment-by-moment focused awareness and openness to the here and now without judgement and with acceptance. It involves deliberate intention to pay attention to momentary experiences. Mindfulness activities are a way to stop the "internal chatter", or self-talk that individuals engage in. As noted, the mind likes to hang around in the past or be preoccupied with the future. Mindfulness helps you focus on the present. Being mindful means identifying one's thoughts and feelings without getting stuck in them. Such dispassionate, non-judgemental sustained awareness have been found to have both psychological and physiological benefits. Mindfulness helps individuals to change that attitude and relationships with their sensations, feelings, thoughts and urges. See the following Website and Workbooks for specific descriptive examples of how to engage in mindfulness.

www.mindful.org

(Google Mindfulness and Addictions and Depression to find a series of Patient Workbooks)

HOW TO DO MINDFULNESS

1. Develop a friendly accepting interest in your present experience. Observe and describe your current emotions and sensations. Live in the present with awareness.

2. Scan your entire body. Notice sensations without trying to change them.

3. Focus attention on your breathing. Inhale and exhale slowly.

Ask yourse f:

> "What is happening right now?"

> "Can I stay with what is happening right now?"

> "Can I a low and accept my feelings and stay in touch with them without reacting to them?"

> "Can I let my feelings go like they are attached to a moving wave or onto a moving cloud?"

> "Can I change my relationship with my feelings and thoughts? If not, how am I reacting to my feelings?"

OTHER SELF-SOOTHING OPTIONS

How can I *distance myself* from my negative emotions by using self-soothing techniques such as:

____ Use meditation or yoga.

____ Use Chinese mindful movement practices such as Tai Chi and Qui Gong.

____ Call or visit a friend.

____ Take my pet dog for a walk.

____ Go for a car ride, walk, bike ride.

____ Listen to music.

____ Do my hobby (paint, woodwork, gardening)

____ Cook, bake.

____ Take a relaxing warm bath; go for a massage.

____ Go for my recovery group meeting.

____ Watch television or movies.

____ Write in my journal or diary.

Give an example of how you have used self-soothing *non-drug taking* activities.

EXERCISE 4
WAYS TO INCREASE YOUR POSITIVE EMOTIONS

As noted in Module III, resilience-engendering positive emotions like optimism, forgiveness, compassion toward others and yourself, gratitude, love, a sense of awe with nature, and the like can *reshape your brain*. Here is a list of examples of ways you can "build and broaden" your positive emotions. Such activities are useful ways to achieve and maintain sobriety and well-being. How many of these activities do you presently use, or have used in the past? When and where have you used them? How did they work? Are there any activities on this list you could consider adding to your Coping Tool Box?

____ 1. Get involved in enjoyable activities.

____ 2. Create a "bucket list" of pleasurable activities you would like to do.

____ 3. Look for the "silver lining" – benefit finding and benefit remembering. Evidence gratitude for things in your life. What gives you hope?

____ 4. Use positive mental imagery of past, present and future activities.

____ 5. Go through a set of pictures with someone and recall positive events in your life.

____ 6. Capitalize upon success. Repeat that which leads to positive emotions – engage in a self-perpetuating "upward spiral".

____ 7. Keep things in perspective. Remember how far you have come and keep reminding yourself of your values and long-term goals.

____ 8. Make a list of things and people for whom you are grateful.

____ 9. Consider your experience with feelings of forgiveness.

"When have you needed forgiveness?"

"When have you experienced forgiveness from someone?"

"When have you offered forgiveness to someone?"

"Have you been able to forgive yourself?"

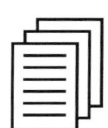

Another way to change your negative emotions is to engage in exercise. Exercise, or what is called Behavioral Activation, has been found to significantly reduce depression and it has a number of other beneficial effects.

Visit the following Website to see how exercise can yield beneficial effects.

www.evanshealth.com/23-and-12-hour

If you are not up to engaging in such strenuous forms of exercise, as Joan Borysenko observes, you can fall back upon the fact that:

Too many people confine their exercise to jumping to conclusions, running up bills, stretching the truth, bending over backwards, lying down on the job, sidestepping responsibility and pushing their luck.

STEPS TO EMOTIONAL WELLNESS

1. Tune into your feelings

2. Name the feelings and rate the level of distress intensity using the SUDs scale

3. Locate these feelings in your body

4. Accept the feelings (Do not try to suppress your feelings)

5. Let your feelings go (melt away, dissipate, be released)

6. When appropriate, share your feelings with someone you trust in a safe place

7. Check the relationship between your thoughts and your feelings

   "When I say this to myself I tend to feel."

   "What am I thinking that makes me feel this way?"

   "What is another way of thinking that could help me manage these feelings?'

   "What can I do to recognize these feelings as soon as they occur?"

   "How can I plan ahead to anticipate situations and people who are likely to trigger these feelings?"

   "Can I stay centered and in control and be aware of the rise and fall of my feelings?"

   "How do these feelings color the way I see things from the past and the present?

"Am I being 'prejudiced' in how I see events and people? Are my feelings acting like blinders and contributing to 'tunnel vision'? How are my feelings influencing how I see the future?"

HOW CAN I CHANGE MY BEHAVIOR IN ORDER TO FEEL BETTER?

"Use my feeling management skills."

"Take a Time Out before the feelings become unmanageable. When the emotions calm down, take a Time In."

"View situations that triggered intense emotions as a set of problems-to-be-solved."

"Ask for help."

DISCUSSION STARTERS FOR MODULE IV

"Addicts don t use on a regular basis because they are addicted, they are addicted because they use a lot, and regularly." Judith Grisel

"No emotion s built to last forever."

"As long as you keep secrets and supress feelings, you're fundamentally vulnerable."

"Embracing patience is the royal road to recovery."

"Imagine being forgiven by someone you respect. Can you now forgive yourself?"

"Survivors' stories have two main themes: Optimism and altruism."

RECOVERY VOICE IV: SURVIVING WEDDING SEASON IN MY FIRST YEAR OF SOBRIETY

In a descriptive article that appeared in the *New York Times* (August 8, 2018), Sarah shared the emotional coping strategies on how she did not drink at seven wedding ceremonies within a 12-month period. Here is a Relapse Prevention Plan worth learning from.

"I was a frequent drinker, wrecked by having anxiety and loneliness."

At the age of 28, Sarah quit drinking with the help of a therapist. How would she deal with the temptations to drink again at these multiple wedding ceremonies — open bar, champagne toasts, social expectations and pressure to drink, and a sadness that she was still unattached?

"My sobriety was a shameful secret that I could not share with anyone."

Here is Sarah's Relapse Prevention Plan, and the emotional coping strategies that she mentally rehearsed and implemented, using her Future Imagery Training and coping procedures.

1. First, she would fill her tumbler with Club Soda, and fill up her plate with food that required two hands to be busy.

2. She decided to be "fun" as a wedding guest, without needing to drink alcohol.

3. She took a Time Out to regroup, by exiting to the bathroom when she felt under pressure to drink again, especially when she felt sorry for herself about still being single. (Sarah was able to talk back to her Amygdala, *not* allowing her emotions to "hijack" her self-regulatory frontal lobes of her brain.)

4. She would text a supportive friend, relating how she was "surviving sober wedding boot camp". (Use of her humor.)

5. She developed a mental schedule, breaking the wedding ceremonies into a set of distinct activities, each with specific behavioral goals filled with self-control strategies and exit plans. By the seventh wedding ceremony, this "game plan" was on autopilot.

6. She also learned to think of herself less and focus on the other guests. *"I learned I did not have to dance with my own inner demons."*

7. She took pride in what she achieved, and most important, she was *"able to remember the wedding ceremony the next day."*

Her game plan was filled with Instead behaviors.

Ways to Strengthen Your Cognitive Coping Tool Box

Exercise 1: Some Facts about Your Thinking Processes

Exercise 2: Thinking Styles of Individuals Who Abuse Substances – "DEFENCE"

Exercise 3: Thinking Traps and "Twisted Thinking"

Exercise 4: Rethinking Skills

Exercise 5: Change Talk and the Languages of Possibilities and Becoming

"Sometimes I do things out of habit, and I do not really stop to think about it. This program made me think about my choices."

As noted, each of us are "homo narrans", or story-tellers. During our whole life we are exposed to other people's stories, and in time we become our own story teller. This module explores the nature of the stories that people who have problems with addictions tell themselves and tell others. Doing the Exercises in this module will increase your awareness and understanding of your thinking processes and co-occurring emotional and behavioral challenges.

As a result, you can develop your own Recovery Stories and accompanying Cognitive Coping Tools.

Exercise 1 begins with a discussion of some facts you should know about your thinking processes and their impact on your feelings and behaviors.

Exercise 2 will consider what is behind the proposition that alcoholism (drug abuse) is *90% thinking and 10% drinking*. What do substance abusing individuals say, and not say to themselves, that contribute to their decision to use?

Exercise 3 will consider the nature of the "thinking traps" and forms of "twisted thinking" that contribute to lapses, relapses and to emotional distress.

Exercise 4 considers the "rethinking skills" you can add to your Coping Tool Box.

Exercise 5 considers Change Talk and the "Language of Possibilities and Becoming" that can contribute to lasting changes, abstinence and well-being.

As a result of completing Module V, you will be able to break the vicious cycle that leads to substance abusing and distressing behavioral patterns. With the assistance of your Treatment Team, not only will you be able to understand, develop and practice these coping skills, but you will be able to "teach" them to others and offer the *reasons* why they are critical in your recovery and in improving your well-being. Moreover, you will be able to anticipate and address, with confidence, any barriers/obstacles that may get in the way.

EXERCISE 1
SOME FACTS ABOUT YOUR THINKING PROCESSES

The concept of "cognition" or thoughts can be divided into three categories.

1. There are *automatic thoughts* or *self-talk*. These may be in the form of words – inner dialogue – with oneself. Sometimes they may be in the form of images and remembrances. These automatic thoughts may be drenched with high emotionality, "hot cognitions", or reflect "hot spots" and "stuck points". In most instances, individuals do *not* question their automatic thoughts and they accept them as "God- given". They may constitute plans, expectations, attributions of responsibility and the like.

    Such automatic thoughts may take a variety of forms. For example, such statements as

    "Yes … but"

    "If … then"

    "In spite of .."

    "On purpose"

    In Exercise 2 we will consider the automatic thoughts of individuals who abuse substances.

2. Cognitions also are made up of *thinking processes* that individuals employ such as:

    a) black and white thinking (all or nothing thinking)

    b) catastrophizing (making a mountain out of a mole hill, blowing things out of proportion)

    c) dwelling on only the negatives

    c) jumping to conclusions and overgeneralizing

    e) "should", "musts", "never", "always" thinking patterns

    f) confirmatory bias in seeking and only accepting information (data) that is consistent with their prior beliefs

("Seek and ye shall find")

Can You Give an Example of Each of These Thought Processes?

3. A third way to view the concept of cognition is as a form of *strongly-held beliefs*, *attitudes* and *values*. Such beliefs can act as a set of "blinders" that color your outlook (being optimistic or pessimistic), and the accompanying feelings you experience. For example,

> Fatalistic beliefs that engender hopelessness and helplessness.

> Beliefs that people are untrustworthy and uncaring.

> Beliefs that one is unlovable, unworthy and is a burden on others.

Individuals may also hold *positive beliefs* that they are resilient and have the ability to "bounce back", and can overcome ongoing adversities.

Which set of beliefs one embraces will determine how effective treatment will be. As the adage goes:

"Our life is what our thoughts make of it."

"We become the stories we tell about ourselves. Beware of the stories you tell yourself and others."

Before we consider the "stories" individuals who abuse substances tell, there is one last important concept to consider. This is what is called Thinking Fast *versus* Thinking Slow. Thinking Fast, or what has been called Type I thinking, reflects an automatic, impulsive, non-reflective reactions. When answering a simple math question such as 2×3, you came up with an answer of 6 right away. No need to calculate or figure out an answer. The answer just pops into your head. Or if you were threatened, your immediate response may be "fight or flight", without stopping to consider options, nor question the nature of the provocation. Or if you are exposed to a salient cue (reminder) to use substances again, your cravings and urges may be immediately triggered.

In contrast, Thinking Slow, or what is called Type II thinking, is designed to be reflective, consequential, and it triggers and involves *frontal lobe-type executive skills*.

"How much is 26×16?"

There is a need to *slow down* and call upon procedural memory and strategies, self-checking and exerting conscious effort to answer this math problem.

Much of the abuse of substances reflects Type I thinking. A major goal of this Patient Workbook is to help individuals develop SMART goals and engage in Type II thinking.

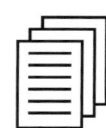

EXERCISE 2
THINKING STYLES OF
INDIVIDUALS WHO ABUSE
SUBSTANCES – "DEFENCE"

"I desperately wish I could stop, and I really mean it, but I can't."

What are the automatic Type I thoughts, thinking processes and beliefs that *sustain* individuals' substance abuse (alcohol, drugs)? As you go through this list, identify any of these thought patterns that you may have used. You can discuss these with your Treatment Team and in your group meetings.

If the alcoholism and drug use is 90% thinking and 10% drinking, then we can ask what goes into the thinking processes that contribute to use? These thought patterns can be summarized using the mnemonic "Defence".[1]

D   Denial processes

E   Entitlement thoughts

F   Fatalistic thoughts

E   Evaluative thoughts about others and about oneself

N   Needs-based thinking processes

C   Illusions of **C**ontrol

E   Expectations of self-satisfying, stimulating experiences

Let's consider how each of these thinking processes contribute to sustaining substance abuse of alcohol and drugs.

The following provides examples of *self-justifying*, *sustaining self-talk* and *self-generated narratives*. This is how you talk yourself out of changing, and provide the reasoning for continuing substance abuse.

1. First, substance abusing individuals may evidence some form of denial or reframe that they have addictive behavior problems:

   "I don't think I have a problem. You are overreacting."

---

[1] Note that in the U.S., the word "Defence" is spelled with an "s". However, in England the word "Defence" is spelled with a "c"., so for the purposes of this acronym, I have chosen the British spelling.

"I don't think I have to change."

"Drinking (substance abuse) is a problem for some people, but not for me."

"I am not an addict, I am only a social drinker."

"I could use and no one would ever know."

"No one in my family was diagnosed as an alcoholic."

2. **Entitlement** thoughts which constitute permission-giving beliefs that they deserve and are entitled ("Earned the right to use"), and moreover, that they have no other options available for obtaining self-deserved pleasures:

"I deserve x."

"I cannot be happy without x."

"I have quit everything else."

"Getting high is the only thing I look forward to."

"I am my own boss and I don't like people telling me how to live."

"It is the only way to be accepted."

3. **Fatalistic** thinking reflects individuals deep-seated feelings of helplessness, powerlessness and uselessness that sustain addictive behaviors:

"I am helpless."

"I feel trapped. This is my only escape."

"I am powerless."

"I lack willpower."

"I am at the mercy of my urges."

"I have hit bottom. What is the use of stopping? I will start again."

"Once an alcoholic, always an alcoholic."

"I am useless."

"I am a complete mess."

"Stopping won't do any good anyway."

"I am stuck in my life. I can never get out of my drug habit."

"I hate myself."

4. **Evaluative** thoughts about others and about oneself which reflect negative views about their relationships with significant others in their lives resulting from feeling marginalized, unsupported and vengeful. Feelings of being rejected, unappreciated and lonely can trigger addictive behaviors.

   "Drinking is my way of getting back at them."

   "No one really cares if I use or not."

   "No one understands me. No one can help me anyway."

   "You can't trust people. In order to be safe, I have to use."

   "No one thinks I am worth saving and I agree."

   "I am a burden on others and they would be better off without me around."

   "I am too tired to continue living."

5. **Need-based** self-statements and beliefs that reflect a tyranny of "shoulds", "needs", "musts" and "cant's". Self-talk that begins with "I need, must, should X", drives the urge to use substances.

   "I need x in order to unwind, avoid withdrawal symptoms, forget, survive."

   "I need x in order to (get some benefits) such as be creative, attractive, sociable and sexy."

   "I must use to have a good life."

   "I can't survive without x."

   "Without x, I can't handle, control, tolerate, cope."

   "Life is unbearable, I have to escape for a while."

   "I need to use x in order to avoid the pain of withdrawal symptoms."

6. **Illusions of control** are held at some level that they can exert control and handle substance abuse behaviors.

   "I can test myself."

   "I am different from others who use."

   "I know how to handle my use."

   "I am more in control of myself, when I use."

   "I can hold my liquor better than others."

© 2020 Donald Meichenbaum, *Treating Individuals with Addictive Disorders: A Strengths-Based Workbook for Patients and Clinicians*, Routledge

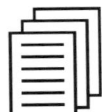

7. **Expectations** of self-satisfying and stimulating experiences as a result of using substances. Such thoughts highlight the expected and perceived physiological, psychological and social benefits of using, especially with others who are also using substances.

"It just feels so good. I love the buzz and the high."

"I need a pick-me-up."

"When I use I feel alive."

"My body needs this to survive."

"If I don't use drugs, I will lose my friends"

"When I use, I have more friends and better sex."

"When I use with others, I can find customers to sell to."

Are there any other examples you can offer of how you convince yourself to continue using? What advice would you have as to how to change these thought patterns and the accompanying addictive behaviors?

EXERCISE 3
THINKING TRAPS AND "TWISTED THINKING"

The first step in changing your behavior is to increase your awareness and interrupt the habitual way one thinks and behaves. There is a need to go off "auto-pilot" (Type I impulsive thinking) and to "mentalize" (use Type II thinking processes).

To mentalize means that people increase their awareness of their thinking processes and their self-talk in the *here and now* and monitor, and alter them, as needed. It means to become an observer of one's own thinking processes, like an outsider.

"I am about to do …"

"I can notice, catch, interrupt …"

"I can think through the consequences of …"

"I have learned to ask myself the questions I usually discuss with my therapist and my sponsor."

A pilot may fly his/her airplane on "auto-pilot", but he/she is constantly aware that should conditions change, there is a need to intervene and take action. Like the pilot, you can go off auto-pilot and take appropriate actions, or mentalize.

THINKING TRAPS AND "TWISTED THINKING"

Individuals who *get stuck* and not able to break old habits tend to fall into "thinking traps" such as ruminating or dwelling on failures and setbacks, "awfulizing", engaging endlessly in "only if" thinking and playing Monday Quarterbacking. They keep asking themselves, over and over "Why" questions for which there are no satisfactory answers. They tend to be perfectionists and berate themselves and see themselves as "losers". They are often their worst "inner critic". They show little or no compassion for themselves and for others.

© 2020 Donald Meichenbaum, *Treating Individuals with Addictive Disorders: A Strengths-Based Workbook for Patients and Clinicians*, Routledge

CAN YOU IDENTIFY THE FOLLOWING "THINKING TRAPS" IN YOUR SELF-TALK?

- Use *polarized thinking* and think in black and white extreme terms. Things are either right or wrong, perfect or horrible, totally safe or unsafe, your either with me or against me.

- "Catastrophize" or "awfulize" – expecting the worst to happen and that you will not be able to handle the situation. Jump to conclusions that you will be a total failure. Focus on only the negative and the worst potential outcomes, so why make the effort to change.

- Be *perfectionistic* and set unrealistic high standards for yourself and others and engage in harsh criticism when standards are not met. Be impatient. Are you too demanding of yourself? There is nothing wrong for striving for excellence, but it is when perfectionism takes over that it can contribute to lapses and relapses.

Perhaps, the impact of thinking traps was best captured by the psychologist Albert Ellis who warned individuals to avoid telling themselves:

"I must/should …"

"People must/should …"

Ellis challenged patients to avoid the *"tyranny of shoulds/musts"*. He cajoled his patients that they not "should on their heads", nor engage in what he called *"must*urbation".

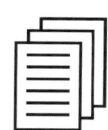

EXERCISE 4
RETHINKING SKILLS

There are a number of *rethinking skills* that you can use to cope with various triggers, urges, cravings, feelings and behaviors of others. The first and most critical step is to *increase your awareness* of when you are falling into a "thinking trap" and engaging in *negative self-talk*. You need to "deautomatize" the act and "mentalize" – using Type II thinking processes. In order to control your reactions and in order to self-regulate you can use SOS coping skills.

S – how to *slow down* and take a break, clear your mind, control impulsive decisions and actions. Listen for "shoulds" and "musts" in your self-talk.

O – *orient*, pay attention to *both* internal and external triggers. Size up the situation – *be a realistic optimist* and *cognitively* **flexible**.

S – *self-check* on your level of stress and choose from your Tool Box of coping skills.

Be prepared to use your back-up strategy. Change your self-talk.

Here is a list of other coping strategies you can employ. Your Treatment Team can review these with you.

1. **Thought Stopping** – When you are having negative thoughts shout "Stop" to yourself. Think of a big red stop sign to help block the thoughts.

2. **Pay Attention to Positives** – Keep track of positive things that have happened. Make a list of things that went well. "Is your glass half empty or half full?" Engage in benefit-finding, benefit remembering, search for the "silver lining".

3. **Challenge Your Thoughts** – In the same way you do *not* believe everything that you hear on television or that you read in the newspaper, why do you *believe* every thought that goes through your head? How can you question, check out, reconsider and reframe your thoughts? *Check out your thoughts*. Be a "thought detective". "I am getting out of my user and victim thinking modes."

4. View Provocations as *problems to be solved*, instead of personal assaults and threats. Become a good problem-solver: Goal–Plan–Do–Check.

5. Use your *relaxation* (tactical breathing) and *mindfulness* skills, namely, ongoing moment-to-moment focused awareness and openness to here and now, without judgement and with acceptance. As noted, mindfulness allows you to stay present and get *grounded* by focusing your attention on the immediate physical environment in the present (where you are and what specifically surrounds you). You can learn to postpone and compartmentalize any worries, your bad feelings and thoughts.

6. Be *self-compassionate toward yourself*, which entails you developing a mental kindness and self-acceptance toward yourself. Develop the ability to self-soothe and be self-nurturing toward yourself. Introduce your "self-compassionate self" to your "self-suffering self".

    a) For example, visit the Website www.self-compassion.org

    b) Envision a good friend came to you with a similar problem that you have. What empathy, compassion and advice might you offer? Could you use the same understanding, kindness and support towards yourself that you would offer your friend? Can you be more patient and non-judgemental toward yourself?

    Individuals high in self-compassion tend to have greater life satisfaction, higher emotional intelligence, greater social connectedness, lower job burnout and higher well-being.

7. Finally, fill your self-talk and story-telling with re-verbs to describe the progress you have made, so far. Be able to tell others in your life, your Treatment Team, your group members, how you are in the midst of:

    RE-framing events

    RE-arranging my life

    RE-setting my priorities

    RE-visiting my past and looking for strengths

    RE-connecting with my spirituality

    RE-discovering the sacred

    RE-wiring my brain

    RE-cruiting chemicals in my brain

    RE-bounding from my trauma history

    RE-linquishing "twisted thinking"

    RE-sisting my cravings/urges

RE-newing relationships

RE-gulating my emotions

RE-thinking my options

RE-building my strengths

RE-building trust

RE-interpreting the situation

RE-working my "story", so it has a better ending

RE-calibrating my Journey of Recovery

When offering these re-verbs, be sure to include examples of how you are doing each activity, and be sure to include the *reasons* why you are engaging in these activities.

As you tell your story be sure to bathe your story and self-talk with action verbs such as "notice", "catch", "interrupt", "plan for", "try out", "question", "fine tune", "self-correct", and other Type II thinking processes. You can enter into a diary examples of your use for:

Re- and actions verbs and *instead* statements. When you attend group meetings or AA meetings listen and count the number of these verbs you hear in other individuals' stories. How many re-verbs and action verbs do you include in your stories? Do you include Change Talk, the Language of Possibilities and Becoming?

EXERCISE 5
CHANGE TALK AND THE LANGUAGES OF POSSIBILITIES AND BECOMING

A major intervention approach to treat individuals with addictive behaviors is called Motivational Interviewing. This is a patient-oriented intervention for enhancing a patient's intrinsic motivation to change by collaboratively exploring his/her decision making processes and ambivalence about changing. See the following Websites for more information on how to increase the likelihood of changing your behavior and achieving your treatment goals.

www.motivationalinterviewing.org

http://ctndisseminationlibrary.org.PDF/146.pdf

A central feature of Motivational Interviewing is to help addicted individuals develop the use of Change Talk. How many of the following type of statements do you include in your self-talk and story-telling? Do your statements reflect the following expressions:

1. Need to change statements

    "I *need* to stop …"

    "I *have to* change …"

    "I *must* …"

    "Something has to change in my life."

2. Desire to change statements"

    "I *really want* to change …"

    "I *wish* I did not use so much."

    "I *would like* to see …"

    "I *want* to reduce …"

    "I *would like* …"

    "I *wish* …"

    "I *hope* …"

3. Ability to change statements

    "I *can* …"

    "I am able to …"

    "I *could* …"

"I would be able to …"

"I think I can cut down on my use."

4. Activation statements like

    "I am *willing to* …"

    "I am *ready to* …"

    "I am *prepared to* …"

    "I am *going to* …"

    "I plan to …"

    "I am considering …"

5. Commitment statements

    "I am going to cut down, maybe even stop using."

    "I want to …"

    "I could …"

    "I will tell _____ about what I am working on."

6. Reasons to change statements

    "I should try to … **because** …"

    "The *reasons* I should … are …"

    "I should *continue* working on …"

    "Things are tough, I cannot afford to …"

In order to achieve lasting sustained change of any behavior, individuals need to "take credit" for their changed behaviors. They have to see the connections between their efforts, their use of specific coping tools and the resultant benefits. Moreover, they have to be able to provide self-generated, unprompted *reasons* why engaging in such change behaviors is critical in their achieving their treatment goals. Their behavior has to be filled with Change Talk and also the Language of Possibilities.

The Language of Possibilities or the Language of Becoming is a type of "future talk" that is solution-focused. The use of such expressions such as "so far" and "as yet" can move you in a direction of change.

"*So far*, things have not gone right for me."

"I have not found a way to stop using, *as yet*."

"*So far*, I have found an *exception* where I was successful in making a change. What I did was …"

"One of the things that gives me hope is …"

© 2020 Donald Meichenbaum. *Treating Individuals with Addictive Disorders: A Strengths-Based Workbook for Patients and Clinicians*, Routledge

Such future talk indicates to others, as well as to oneself, that there are potential solutions to be found down the road.

In your efforts to be optimistic there is a need to be a Realistic Optimist who can see past failures and future challenges, but can be cognitively flexible to size up a situation, staying open to future possibilities.

As the observation goes:

The Pessimist complains about the wind.

The Optimist expects the wind to change.

The Realistic Optimist adjusts the sail.

As noted, another way to engage in future talk that is realistically optimistic is to convey that you are on a journey to recovery, abstinence and well-being. A journey metaphor is a useful way to convey that you have a destination or goal in mind, although the destination may change along the way. On your personal journey you may expect detours, setbacks and surprises, but that you have the *grit* to continue on. In order to navigate your personal journey, you have an internal GPS (this Patient Workbook) that will help you.

Individuals have developed ways to remind themselves and access such Change Talk by putting their self-talk on their cellphone, IPAD, computers and in the form of flash cards, and the like. The following list of Coping Control Beliefs and Change Talk have been used by individuals. From this list choose some examples (or add others) that you can use to redirect your narrative.

EXAMPLES OF COPING CONTROL BELIEFS AND CHANGE TALK

I can't change the past, but I have a life worth living.

I might not always tell the truth, but my actions don't lie.

I role play coping scenes in my mind.

I learned that it is okay to be uncomfortable. I need to challenge myself every day.

I cultivate a spiritual connection on a daily basis.

I listen for the strength in my inner voice.

I tell myself that I am not my trauma nor my addiction, but I learned how they go together.

If I stop using now, I can show myself and others that I am stronger than the drugs.

Walking away from alcohol is the same as walking toward saving my marriage.

I must seek drug-free friends when I feel badly.

I do not need drugs to have fun (be sociable, creative, sexy).

My life will improve without drugs.

I can cope with unpleasant emotions without booze.

Even if I sip up, I don't have to continue using.

A lapse is not equivalent to a failure or a full relapse.

I can experience a high without using x.

I am less likely to make good decisions and keep myself safe when I am high.

Getting high could get me in trouble and mess with my head.

I can put the problem of addiction behind me.

There are multiple pathways to change and I can find the best pathway for me.

Remember that small changes in language, self-talk and story-telling can open new possibilities for future change.

HOPE BEGETS HOPE

Consider one last example of how Change Talk can predict treatment outcomes.

Researchers at the University of British Columbia in Canada conducted a study in which they asked alcoholics the following questions:

"Please think about the last time you drank alcohol and felt bad about yourself as a result. This might be a time when you slipped from your sobriety. Please describe in as much detail as possible what happened, how it made you feel, and what you did in response to this event?"

"When was the last time you were tempted to use and did not give into (resisted) the temptation? How did you handle the situation?"

How the alcoholics answered these questions predicted their long-term recovery. If their answers included statements reflecting self-control and renewed motivation and efforts of self-improvement, they were more likely to remain substance free and abstinent. For example, consider how they answered these questions.

"I can see what I did was wrong the last time and I can learn from it."

"My obsession with using lifted and I feel relieved."

"I have resisted my cravings before and I can do it again."

"My cravings in the past have passed and these will too."

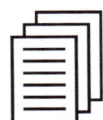

"Having a craving is not a commandment to use."

The expression of such beliefs reflect the alcoholics' commitment to maintain sobriety and proved helpful in achieving abstinence. The reasons people offer themselves and others play a powerful role in developing the coping skills to control substance abuse.

Yet, another way to re-author your life story and to develop a Sobriety Script is to engage in *writing exercises* or some form of *journaling*. Research has demonstrated that having individuals express their feelings by writing about them on a regular basis serves several very therapeutic functions. These include helping individuals:

1. make sense of negative events and accompanying negative feelings that they have experienced;

2. develop a more coherent account with a beginning, middle and ends of what happened, instead of getting stuck on "hot spots" and "stuck points" and ruminating or dwelling on some events;

3. develop a perspective considering the viewpoint of others;

4. become a better "detective" in your ability to conduct an analysis of what contributed to lapses and relapse. (Conduct your Clock analysis – 12, 3, 6 and 9 o'clock);

5. engage in non-negative thinking and include in your written account the "rest of the story" of what you have done in the past that reflects resilience and strengths. Some individuals have written what they call "rainy day" letters to themselves. They write a letter to themselves when they are feeling strong and hopeful indicating strengths and resolution. This letter can be read when you feel the need. This letter can remind you that you have survived "bad days" in the past and how you accomplished this in your written or oral accounts. *Count* the number of times you include:

    a. the word *instead* and examples;

    b. the number of re- verbs, action verbs, with examples;

    c. the presence of Change Talk and the Language of Possibilities ("so far", "as yet");

    d. a list of pros and cons about not wanting to change and the *reasons* for changing.

Remember that "the stories we tell ourselves and others function to influence the life we live. We are lived by the stories we tell."